THE USE OF HYPNOSIS IN SURGERY AND ANESTHESIOLOGY

THE USE OF HYPNOSIS IN SURGERY AND ANESTHESIOLOGY

Psychological Preparation of the Surgical Patient

By

Lillian E. Fredericks, M.D.

Diplomat of the American Board of Anesthesiology
Diplomat of the American Board of Medical Hypnosis

Contributors

Frederick J. Evans, Ph.D.
Daniel P. Kohen, M.D., F.A.A.P.
Patrick McCarthy, M.B.Ch.B., DRCOG.
Karen N. Olness, M.D.

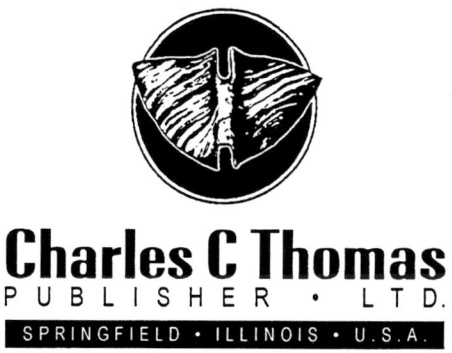

Charles C Thomas
PUBLISHER · LTD.
SPRINGFIELD · ILLINOIS · U.S.A.

Published and Distributed Throughout the World by

CHARLES C THOMAS • PUBLISHER, LTD.
2600 South First Street
Springfield, Illinois 62704

This book is protected by copyright. No part of
it may be reproduced in any manner without
written permission from the publisher.

©2001 by CHARLES C THOMAS • PUBLISHER, LTD.

ISBN 0-398-07128-4 (cloth)
ISBN 0-398-07129-2 (paper)

Library of Congress Catalog Card Number: 00-060769

With THOMAS BOOKS *careful attention is given to all details of manufacturing
and design. It is the Publisher's desire to present books that are satisfactory as to their
physical qualities and artistic possibilities and appropriate for their particular use.*
THOMAS BOOKS *will be true to those laws of quality that assure a good name
and good will.*

*Printed in the United States of America
TL-R-3*

Library of Congress Cataloging-in-Publication Data

Fredericks, Lillian E.
　The use of hypnosis in surgery and anesthesiology: psychological preparation of the surgical patient / by Lillian E. Fredericks; contributors, Frederick J. Evans . . . [et al.].
　　p. cm.
Includes bibliographical references and index.
ISBN 0-398-07128-4 (cloth)–ISBN 0-398-07129-2 (pbk.)
　1. Hypnotism in surgery. 2. Hypnotism in surgery–Psychological aspects. 3. Anesthesia–Psychological aspects. I. Evans, Frederick J. II. Title.

RD85.H9 F74 2000
617'.05–dc21

00-060769

Erika Fromm and Karen Olness urged me to document, in the form of a book, my use of hypnosis as an anesthesiologist preparing patients for anesthesia and surgery. I am very proud of their trust in me. Erika always encouraged me when I was overwhelmed with the enormity of the task and she listened patiently to my reading all the chapters to her. Her criticism and her suggestions were very valuable to me. I am eternally grateful to her and I dedicate this volume to her.

CONTRIBUTORS

Frederick J. Evans, Ph.D., President, Pathfinders: Consultants in Human Behavior, Lawrenceville, New Jersey; Chief Psychologist: Pain Management Service, Medical Center of Princeton, New Jersey. The Back Rehabilitation Center, Hamilton and Princeton, New Jersey, Pain Care Institute, Philadelphia, Pennsylvania. Address: 736 Lawrence Road, Lawrenceville, New Jersey.

Lillian E. Fredericks, M.D., ABMH., retired from the Department of Anesthesiology at the Hospital of the University of Pennsylvania, in Philadelphia. She is a Diplomat of the American Society of Anesthesiology, Diplomat of the American Society of Medical Hypnosis and Fellow of the American Society of Clinical Hypnosis, Clinical and Experimental Hypnosis, International Society of Hypnosis and The Swedish Society of Hypnosis. Address: 3360 South Ocean Blvd., Apt. 3HS, Palm Beach, Florida 33480.

Daniel P. Kohen, M.D., F.A.A.P., Director Behavioral Pediatrics Program, Professor Department of Pediatrics and Family Practice and Community Health, University of Minnesota. Address: Behavioral Pediatrics Program, University Specialists Suite 804, 606 24th Avenue, South Minneapolis, Minnesota 55454.

Patrick McCarthy, M.B.Ch.B., DRCOG, MRNZCGP, received a Diploma of the Royal College of Obstetricians and Gynecologists. Member of the Royal New Zealand College of General Practitioners, Diplomat New Zealand Society of Clinical Hypnosis, President of New Zealand Society of Hypnosis, The Milton H. Erickson Institute of Wellington, New Zealand. Address: 9th Floor, CMC Building, 89 Courtenay Place, Wellington, New Zealand.

Karen N. Olness, M.D., Professor of Pediatrics, Family Medicine and International Health, Case Western Reserve University, Cleveland, Ohio; Director Rainbow Center for International Child Health; Director International Child Health Training Fellowship and Co-Director Behavioral Pediatrics Training Fellowship. Address: 2042 E. 115th Street, Cleveland, Ohio 44106.

FOREWORD

At the turn of the last century, the anesthetic death rate from ether and chloroform was one in four hundred at university hospitals. Then Alice Magaw (1906) reported over 14,000 consecutive anesthetics without a death, and it became clear why you should go to the Mayo clinic for elective surgery—you didn't die under anesthesia!* Her article tells why. Her father, who used hypnosis, had taught her the art of suggestion, and once the abdomen was open and surgery begun, she shut off the ether and suggested nice things to the patient until she had to give ether again to allow closure of the wound. The patients received very little ether during a major procedure.

Lillian Fredericks has brought together in this book the things we have learned in a century of progress. Her fellow anesthetists have made it their goal to alleviate, prevent, and control both pain and suffering. She uses hypnosis as an integral part of this effort, and describes how it enhances all aspects of pain control. There are chapters on hypnosis as the sole anesthetic, as an adjunct to chemical anesthesia, and in conjunction with regional anesthesia. She takes us to the intensive care ward and the emergency room where pain and suffering are rampant, and tells us how to assuage fear and suffering with soothing suggestions. She has enlisted the collaboration of outstanding experts on hypnosis and human misery – Fred Evans, Dan Kohen, Pat McCarthy, and Karen Olness.

My own experience as a surgeon trained in hypnosis has made me wonder if the trance state in the human may not be analogous to the protective states we see throughout nature. The tetanus spore is almost indestructible, able to withstand heat, cold, and chemicals, but in its vegetative state, it is susceptible to antibiotics and oxygen. The amebic cyst is untouchable by medicines, but in its active trophozoite state,

---

Magaw, A. (1906). A review of over fourteen thousand surgical anaesthesias. *Surgery, Gynecology & Obstetrics, 3*:795–797.

there are many antibiotics that are effective against it. Plants and trees that are dormant in winter can be transplanted, pruned, and grafted, but in summer when the sap is rising, they are likely to die if this is done. Bears and squirrels hibernate, and experience marked diminution in their metabolic needs. I wonder if hypnosis in humans is similar to the protective states we see in lower forms of life, and if so, then shouldn't it be an adjunct for every patient undergoing general anesthesia and the trauma of surgery?

Dabney M. Ewin, M.D.
Clinical Professor of Surgery and Psychiatry
Tulane University Medical School
Clinical Professor of Psychiatry
Louisiana State University Medical School

PREFACE

The definition of Hypnosis by the American Psychological Association is: Hypnosis is a procedure, in which a therapist or researcher suggests that a client or subject experience changes in sensations, perceptions, thoughts, or behaviors (Kirsch 1994). This only describes the procedure (possibly the induction) but not the subtle complexities of feeling, perceiving, thinking and/or behavior, which is the essence of hypnosis. Hypnosis is not a one-way street; it is an interactive experience. Linden (1997) describes it so well: "It is not what one does to another, but a process that takes place through the relationship of healer to healee." Hilgard (1973b) postulated the domain of hypnosis comprehensively and Bowers (1983) states: ". . . hypnosis involves absorptive and dissociative experiences that are less visible than hypnotic suggestibility per se, but they are perhaps even more important in determining the domain of hypnosis." This book will not concentrate on the procedure of hypnosis (the induction process) but on the experience and the intrinsic value of this medical modality. In some of the following chapters, it will be shown that a hypnotic induction is often not necessary for patients to slip into this state of altered consciousness, during which suggestibility increases to a great extent. It is awe inspiring to observe what the human mind can accomplish when guided by appropriate hypnotic suggestions and to observe psychological and physiological changes which follow.

Hypnosis has been used for many centuries in many different ways and under many different names. In ancient times, there were sleep temples in Egypt, and in Greece; Aesculapian rituals were practiced and Delphic Oracles were consulted. There was Animal Magnetism practiced by Franz Anton Mesmer (1734-1815). The Marquis de Puysegur (1751-1825) described artificial somnambulism; James Braid (1795-1860) named the phenomenon "Hypnosis," although Gravitz and Gerton (1984) question this and believe that it was used by Baron d'Hnin de Cuvillers and Mialle in 1820. Gravitz (1997) also believes that Charles Lafontaine, a French mesmerist "might be the link between Braid and the much earlier sources," and finally, James Esdaile (1808-1859), a British surgeon, used what might be called "Hypnoanaesthesia" for 300 major cases and 80 percent of his surgical patients felt no pain.

Since that time, hypnosis has been used by many professionals in all kinds of specialties with good results in all fields of medicine. A few unusual applications might be of interest: Abraham (1971) was able to help 13 out of 17 patients to conceive with the use of hypnosis, after they had tried for many years unsuccessfully. Cheek (1995) stopped preterm labor via the telephone, Levitan (1992) used hypnosis extensively with cancer patients, and Ewin (1986a) stopped burns from progressing and (1992a) removed warts without leaving a scar. Spiegel (1993) used hypnosis to treat posttraumatic stress disorders. Crasilneck (1997) discussed a patient terminally ill with metastatic cancer, undergoing hypnotherapy, resulting in complete remission for 11 years.

Research in laboratories and in clinics has flourished because in 1955 the British Medical Association and in 1958 the American Medical Association declared hypnosis a qualifying medical modality. In 1949, the American Society of Clinical and Experimental Hypnosis was founded by Jerome Schneck and Jack Watkins and in 1957 the American Society of Clinical Hypnosis followed. A lot of research has been done and published by their members. Hilgard, at the Stanford Laboratory of Hypnosis, has been in the forefront of research in hypnosis, Bowers (1983, p 30). The *Journal of the American Society of Clinical and Experimental Hypnosis* was first published in 1953 with Milton Kline as the founding editor. The *Journal of the American Society of Clinical Hypnosis* was started in 1959, and David Cheek was one of the first to publish observations and research in the field of hypnosis in surgery, launching a vast body of literature on this subject. Frankel (1987) summarized significant developments in hypnosis which have occurred since that time. Now, thirteen years later, the art and science of hypnosis has matured and progressed, and it is regrettable that medical schools and residency programs in universities still do not include the teaching of hypnosis in their curriculum. A national survey of training programs in hypnosis Walling, Baker & Dot (1998) found that only 36 percent of APA accredited programs offered such courses, many of them on an elective basis. Australia and the Netherlands have national training models (Dane & Kessler 1998), and there is a great need to establish an integrated program of training in the United States. Oster (1998) describes such a formal, integrated curriculum in clinical hypnosis, which is given at the Adler School of Professional Psychology.

There have been many theories to explain the phenomena of hypnosis. Presently there are two prominent theories, mainly differing in paradigms: the neo-dissociation or special process theory, proposed by Hilgard (1973a,1991), notable proponents of which are Orne (1977), Fromm (1977), Shor (1979), and Bowers as quoted by Woody and Farvolden (1992); and the socio-psychological or cognitive-behavioral theory, proposed by Barber (1969), Coe (1989, 1992), Spanos (1991, 1992), and Lynn and Sivec (1992). The main difference between these researchers is that "special process researchers (altered state theory) tend to view hypnotic responses, at least in highly responsive Ss, as something that "happens" to them rather than something that they are "doing" (Coe, 1992), whereas socio-psychological researchers view hypnotic responsiveness "as Ss purposeful, goal-directed strivings to present themselves as hypnotized" (Coe, 1992, p 229). Proponents of the altered state theory believe, that following a hypnotic induction, good subjects will dissociate and become more suggestible and more responsive to suggestion (Lynn, Rhue, & Weekes, 1989). King and Council (1998) showed that one group of high dissociators was responding to amnesia suggestions in a nonintentional mode, whereas other good hypnotic subjects showed more intentional responding to amnesia suggestions. Kihlstrom (1997) summarizes it so beautifully, "Hypnosis is a complex phenomenon, simultaneously a social interaction, with hypnotist and subject interacting in a larger socio-cultural context, and a state of altered consciousness, involving basic cognitive mechanisms underlying perception, memory, and thought." Barabasz (1997) reports that, "Recent EEG research establishes hypnosis as a specialized attentional state which is highly sensitive to formulation of hypnotic instructions."

The history of hypnosis in general is fascinating, and Gauld (1992) has published a very complete compendium. Several authors have reviewed the literature dealing with the use of hypnosis to decrease the stress and anxiety connected with surgery. The most recent and complete reviews were published by Evans and Stanley (1990) and by Blankfield (1991).

Sobel and Ornstein (1996) reported, "In an analysis of over 190 studies of psychological preparation for surgery, 80 percent of the patients showed significant benefits: quicker recovery, fewer complications, less postsurgical pain, less need for pain medication, less anxiety and depression, and an average of 1.5 days less in hospitals." The cost effectiveness of this alone might impress people who are involved in today's healthcare system, not to speak about all the advantages we can afford our patients.

The chapters written by me are a combination of my own experience of using hypnosis as an adjunct in my practice of anesthesiology, the practice of other anesthesiologists, as well as many bibliographic references, using hypnosis not only for the control of pain, anxiety, stress, and apprehension but for many other problems. The work of Esther Bartlett (1966, 1971) and many personal communications with her as well as the work of Bertha Rodger (1961) have influenced my thinking about and my practice of using hypnosis routinely. Because the use of hypnosis in surgery and anesthesiology is multifaceted, I searched for other physicians and psychologists to supplement my knowledge and practice. I was fortunate to find four contributors, all of whom are outstanding in their field, and I thank them for their contributions.

The purpose of the book is to stimulate physicians to explore the vast capabilities of the human mind, when it is working together with the body, and with the help of the unconscious, to accept hypnotic suggestions. I hope it will invite them to use this modality in their own practice.

Medical hypnosis is not fixed and rigid but dynamic and ever changing, as human beings and their needs change. How different is the art and science of using hypnosis now, compared to the time of Mesmer (1734-1815). Two centuries ago, Mesmer, believing in animal magnetism, helped and healed thousands of people, and Esdaile (1808-1859) was able to relieve the excruciating pain during major surgery. What will happen to the practice of hypnosis during the next century, as our knowledge of the workings of the human mind and the unconscious increases, with the help of the research being done all over the world, mainly by psychologists. Elkins and Wall (1996) found that 85 percent of practitioners in a group of 400 physicians, affiliated with a large university health science center, expressed an interest in hypnosis education. However, only a small percentage of physicians are actually using hypnosis in their practice. This is probably due to various misconceptions among lay people as well as professionals;

most commonly, the belief that it takes "so much extra time." The fact is that the use of hypnosis facilitates and actually shortens the length of time to achieve a desired goal (Fredericks, 1980).

Prior to using hypnosis, I interviewed, observed and listened very carefully to all my patients during the preoperative visit. I wanted to find out what they experience, what causes their anxiety, apprehension, and occasionally, near panic. I asked myself what I could do to help them to overcome their fears and thereby get their psychology and physiology into a more stable and more normal condition. During these years of searching, I came to the conclusion that with the use of hypnosis and hypnotic techniques, we can inform patients and make appropriate suggestions to reduce their anxiety and change their perception of the impending procedures, while they are in a very vulnerable and receptive state.

For the following 21 years, I have been using the techniques described in this book for all my patients requiring surgery, both minor and major. I also taught a course in hypnosis to residents and some staff members in the department of anesthesiology, at the Hospital of the University of Pennsylvania, in Philadelphia.

From the beginning of my practice of using hypnosis in conjunction with treating various problems, I have taught self-hypnosis to all my patients, usually in the first or second visit. The importance of active participation of the patient to develop "psychological conditions for therapeutic effects" (Price, 1996) is now recognized by most practitioners and researchers. I have used this concept intuitively throughout the years I have been using hypnosis as an adjunct to various therapeutic interventions. The list is vast.

We now have good documentation that human beings are capable of regulating many autonomic functions, such as blood pressure, heart rate and rhythm, peripheral temperature, etc., which we thought were not under voluntary control. With appropriate suggestions under hypnosis, we can facilitate and augment these responses. As one observes the good results patients are able to achieve with the use of self-hypnosis, one becomes more and more confident and impressed by the power of suggestions made while patients are in hypnosis. Because of the excellent research, which has been done during the past 30 years or more, we now have scientific proof that hypnosis truly facilitates the unconscious acceptance of suggestions, and patients are able to influence not only psychological, but also physiological parameters on their own, using this modality. Among others, Barber (1996) states that the hypnotic state facilitates the analgesia induced by suggestion. One can assume that the same holds true for other suggestions made during hypnosis.

We now have excellent, well-controlled studies to show the effect of suggestions made to patients, in a hypnotic state, such as the control of heart rate and rhythm (Bleeker, 1973a and b), the reduction of blood lost during surgery (Bennett, Benson & Kuicken, 1986), to stop the bleeding by hemophiliacs (Frederichs, 1967), the rapidity of healing and lack of complications, and the enhancement of the immune system (Hall, 1983 & Dillon, Minchoff & Baker, 1985) to name just a few. It is very rewarding to get confirmation from clinicians and experimentalists alike. Researchers in the laboratory and clinicians must work together, observing and experimenting with hypnosis, in order to detect all potentials of the mind-body connection. Covino (1997) published an excellent article on this subject, making several suggestions for integration and collaboration among researchers and clinicians. It is in this spirit that this volume is written and hopefully it will stimulate clinicians to do well-controlled clinical studies, using their vast experience, accumulated during treating their patients.

REFERENCES

Abraham, H.A. (1971). The use of hypnosis in sterility. *Journal of the Albert Einstein Medical Center, 19*(2), 65–67

Barabasz, A. (1997). Hypnosis, pain and attentional processes. 14th International Congress of Hypnosis, San Diego, CA.

Barber J. (1996): *Hypnosis and suggestion in the treatment of pain: A Clinical Guide.* New York, London: W.W. Norton, 88.

Barber, T.X. (1969). *Hypnosis: A scientific approach.* New York: Van Nostrand Reinhold.

Bartlett, E.E. (1966). Polypharmacy versus hypnosis in surgical patients. *Pacific Medicine and Surgery, 74,* 109–112.

Bartlett, E.E. (1971). The use of hypnotic techniques without Hypnosis per se for temporary stress. *American Journal of Clinical Hypnosis, 13:* 273–278.

Bennett, H.L., Benson D.R., & Kuiken, D.A. (1986). Preoperative instructions for decreased bleeding during spine surgery. *Anesthesiology, 65*(3A), A245.

Blankfield, R.P. (1991). Suggestion, relaxation, and hypnosis as adjuncts in the care of surgery patients: A review of the literature. *American Journal of Clinical Hypnosis, 33*(3), 172–186.

Bleecker, E.R., & Engel, B.T. (1973b). Learned control of cardiac rate and cardiac conduction in the Wolff-Parkinson-White syndrome. *New England Journal of Medicine, 288,* 560-562.

Bleecker, E.R., & Engel, B.T. (1973a). Learned control of ventricular rate in patients with atrial fibrillation. *Psychosomatic Medicine, 35*(2), 161-175.

Bowers, K.S. (1983). *Hypnosis for the seriously interested.* New York, London: W.W. Norton.

Cheek, D.B. (1995). Early use of psychotherapy in prevention of preterm labor: The application of hypnosis and ideomotor techniques with women carrying twin pregnancies. *Pre- and Perinatal Psychology Journal, 10*(1), 5-19.

Coe, W.C. (1989) Hypnosis: The role of sociopolitical factors in a paradigm clash. In N.P. Spanos & J.F. Chaves (Eds.), *Hypnosis: The cognitive-behavioral perspective* (p. 418-436), Buffalo, NY: Prometheus.

Coe, W.C. (1992) Hypnosis: Wherefore art thou? *International Journal of Clinical and Experimental Hypnosis, 40*(4), 219-237.

Covino, N.A. (1997). The integration of clinical and experimental work. *The International Journal of Clinical and Experimental Hypnosis, 45*(2), 109-125.

Crasilneck, H.B. (1997). The use of hypnosis in the control of pain. 14th International Congress of Hypnosis, San Diego, CA.

Dane, J.R., & Kessler, R. (1998). Future developments in professional hypnosis training: Review and critique of available training with consideration for development of a nationally coordinated program. *American Journal of Clinical Hypnosis, 41*:1, 38-54.

Dillon, M., Minchoff, B. & Baker, K.H. (1985). Positive emotional states and enhancement of the immune system. *International Journal of Psychiatry in Medicine, 15*:1, 13-18.

Elkins, G.R., & Wall, V.J. (1996). Medical referrals for hypnotherapy: Opinions of physicians, residents, family practice outpatients, and psychiatry outpatients. *American Journal of Clinical Hypnosis, 38*(4), 254-262.

Evans, B.J., & Stanley, R.O. (1990). Psychological interventions for coping with surgery: A review of hypnotic techniques. *Australian Journal of Clinical and Experimental Hypnosis, 18*(2), 97-105.

Ewin, D.M. (1986a). The effect of hypnosis and mental set on major surgery and burns. *Psychiatric Annals, 16*(2), 115-118.

Ewin, D.M., (1992a). Hypnotherapy for warts (veruca vulgaris): 41 consecutive cases with 33 cures. *American Journal of Clinical Hypnosis, 35*(1), 1-10.

Frankel, F.H. (1987). Significant developments in medical hypnosis the past 25 years. *The American Journal of Clinical and Experimental Hypnosis, 35,* 231-247.

Fredericks, L.E. (1967). The use of hypnosis in hemophilia. *American Journal of Clinical Hypnosis, 10*(1), 52-55.

Fredericks, L.E. (1980). The value of teaching hypnosis in the practice of anesthesiology. *The International Journal of Clinical and Experimental Hypnosis, 28*(1), 6-14.

Fromm, E. (1977). An ego-psychological theory of altered states of consciousness. *International Journal of Clinical and Experimental Hypnosis, 25,* 372-387.

Gauld, A. (1992). *A history of hypnotism.* Cambridge: Cambridge University Press, XVII.

Gravitz, M.A., (1997). First uses of "Hypnotism" nomenclature: A historical record. *Hypnos, 24*(1), 42–46.

Gravitz, M.A., & Gerton, M.I. (1984). Origins of the term hypnotism prior to Braid. *American Journal of Clinical Hypnosis, 27,* 107–110.

Hall, H.H. (1983). Hypnosis and the immune system: A review with implications for cancer and the psychology of healing. *American Journal of Clinical Hypnosis, 25,* 92–103.

Hilgard, E.R. (1973a). A neo-dissociation theory of pain reduction in hypnosis. *Psychology Revue, 80,* 396–411.

Hilgard, E.R. (1973b). The domain of hypnosis. *American Psychologist, 28,* 972–982.

Hilgard, E.R. (1991). A neodissociation interpretation of hypnosis. In S. J. Lynn & J.W. Rhue (Eds.), *Theories of hypnosis: Current models and perspectives,* pp 83–104. New York: Guilford.

Kihlstrom, J.F. (1997). Convergence in understanding hypnosis? Perhaps, but perhaps not quite so fast. *The International Journal Clinical and Experimental Hypnosis, 45*(3), 324–332.

King, B.J., & Council, J.R. (1998). Intentionality during hypnosis: An ironic process analysis. *Internetional Journal of Clinical and Experimental Hypnosis, 46*(3), 295–313.3.

Kirsch, I. (1994). APA definition; Description of hypnosis: Defining hypnosis for the public. *Contemporary Hypnosis, 11,* 142–143.

Levitan, A.A. (1992). The use of hypnosis with cancer patients. *Psychiatric medicine: Hypnosis and its clinical applications in psychiatry and medicine,* in Moshe S. Torem (Guest Ed.), 10(1), 119–131.

Linden, J.H. (1997). On the art of hypnotherapy with women: Journeys to the birthplace of belief and other recipes for life. *Hypnosis, 24*(3), 138–147.

Lynn, S.J., & Sivec, H. (1992). The hypnotizable subject as a creative problem-solving agent. In E. Fromm & M.R. Nash (Eds.), *Contemporary hypnosis research,* pp. 292–333. New York: Guilford.

Lynn, S.L., Rhue, J.W., & Weekes, J.R. (1989). Hypnosis and experienced non-volition: A social-cognitive integrative model. In N.P. Spanos & J.F. Chaves (Eds.). *Hypnosis: The cognitive-behavioral perspective.* Buffalo, NY: Prometheus.

Orne, M.T. (1977). The construct of hypnosis: Implications of the definition for research and practice. *Annals of the New York Academy of Science, 296,* 14–33.

Oster, M.I. (1998). A Graduate school curriculum in clinical Hypnosis. *American Journal of Clinical Hypnosis,41*:1, 65–74.

Price, D.D. (1996). In J. Barber, *Hypnosis and suggestions in the treatment of Pain.* New York, London: W.W. Norton & Co.

Rodger, B.P. (1961). The art of preparing the patient for anesthesia. *Anesthesiology, 22*(4), 548–554.

Shor, R.E., (1979). A phenomological method for the measurement of variables important to an understanding of hypnosis. In E. Fromm & R.E. Shor (Eds.), *Hypnosis: Development in research and new perspectives* (Rev. 2nd ed.) Hawthorne, NY: Aldine, pp. 105–135.

Sobel, D.S., & Ornstein, R. (1996). *The healthy mind, healthy body handbook.* Los Altos, CA.: DRX, p 259.

Spanos, N.P. (1991). A sociocognitive approach to hypnosis. In S.J. Lynn & J.W. Rhue (Eds.), *Theories of hypnosis: Current models and perspectives,* pp. 324–361. New York: Guilford.

Spanos, N.P., & Coe, W.C. (1992). A social-psychological approach to hypnosis. In E. Fromm & M.R. Nash (Eds.), *Contemporary hypnosis research* (pp. 102–130). New York: Guilford.

Spiegel, D. (1993). Hypnosis in the treatment of posttraumatic stress disorders. In J.W. Rhue, S.J. Lynn, & I. Kirsch (Eds.), *Handbook of clinical hypnosis.* Washington, D.C.: American Psychological Association, 493–507.

Walling, D.P., Baker, J.M., & Dot, S.G. (1998). Scope of hypnosis education in academia: Results of a national Survey. *International Journal of Clinical & Experimental Hypnosis, 46* (2), 150–156.

Woody, E., & Farvolden, P. (1992): Dissociation in hypnosis and frontal executive function. *American Journal of Clinical Hypnosis, 40*:3, 206–216.

INTRODUCTION

The use of hypnosis in surgery and anesthesia does not seem to have any influence on operative mortality. However, hypnosis and hypnotic techniques teach patients a way to alter their body's reaction to the insult of surgery and all the poisons we use to create unconsciousness. The use of hypnosis alters the psychological state of the patient which, in turn, influences the psychological and physiological reaction to the insult. This book describes in detail how to teach patients, in just a few minutes, what they can do to accomplish this. It also lists the vast amount of research which has been done to document these physiological changes, that seem to be the result of the use of hypnosis.

ACKNOWLEDGMENTS

The contributors to this book have made it complete and their expertise has enriched its quality. I am very grateful for their contributions. I know that they are very busy in their own practices and I appreciate their acceptance of my invitation. Daniel Kohen was always encouraging, available, and willing to give me good advice, especially during the frustrating time while searching for a publisher. Esther Bartlett and her friend Bertha Rodger were pioneers in the use of psychological preparation of the surgical patient. I am also deeply grateful to my friend Sylvia Haymes who made the proofreading much less of a chore.

CONTENTS

	Page
Preface	xi
Introduction	xxi

Chapter

1. AN INTRODUCTION TO HYPNOSIS—*Frederick J. Evans* 3
2. HYPNOSIS AND THE MANAGEMENT 31
   OF CHRONIC PAIN—*Frederick J. Evans*
3. HYPNOSIS IN CONJUNCTION WITH 57
   CHEMICAL ANESTHESIA—*Lillian E. Fredericks*
4. HYPNOSIS IN CONJUNCTION 94
   WITH REGIONAL ANESTHESIA—*Lillian E. Fredericks*
5. HYPNOSIS AS THE SOLE 99
   ANESTHETIC—*Lillian E. Fredericks*
6. HYPNOSIS IN THE INTENSIVE 119
   CARE UNIT—*Lillian E. Fredericks*
7. HYPNOSIS IN THE EMERGENCY 126
   ROOM—*Lillian E. Fredericks*
8. HYPNOSIS IN PEDIATRIC SURGERY—*Daniel P. Kohen* 138
9. HYPNOSIS IN OBSTETRICS AND 163
   GYNECOLOGY—*Patrick McCarthy*
10. PERSPECTIVES FROM 212
    PHYSICIAN-PATIENTS—*Karen N. Olness*

Epilogue—*Lillian E. Fredericks*	223
Author Index	225
Subject Index	231
About the Author	241

THE USE OF HYPNOSIS IN
SURGERY AND ANESTHESIOLOGY

Chapter 1

HYPNOSIS: AN INTRODUCTION

FREDERICK J. EVANS

It is generally agreed that the modern history of hypnosis dates back to the late 18th century with Mesmer. However, it was the Scottish physician, James Esdaile (1850), who first documented the use of hypnosis in the control of pain. Just prior to the development of chemical anesthesia, Esdaile was using hypnosis widely in India as the only form of anesthesia for amputations, tumor removals, and other complex surgical procedures. Overlooked in Esdaile's reports was the finding that most of the patients survived surgery! This finding was especially compelling because at that time most surgical patients died because of hemorrhage, shock, and infection.

As well as controlling surgical pain, hypnosis may have led to autonomic and immunologic effects that minimized the complications of the surgical techniques of the time. Esdaile's surprising result is only now beginning to attract research interest. Clinical reports document that hypnosis has been used as an effective technique to control chronic pains (Sacerdote, 1970; Hilgard & Hilgard, 1975). Only a few studies demonstrate the value of hypnosis in hemophiliac (Dubin & Shapiro, 1974) and cancer patients (Domangue & Margolis, 1983), and when used preoperatively or during surgery to reduce bleeding volume and time (Bennet, Benson & Kuiken, 1986) or to facilitate postoperative recovery measures (Enquist, Konow & Bysted, 1996), as well as reducing pain and postoperative medication (Turner & Chapman, 1982).

---

*I wish to thank George Strobel for his valuable suggestions, and to Blanche Anderson for her expert editorial help I especially want to thank the many teachers and workshop leaders from many countries who have taught me what I know and understand about hypnosis.

The aim of this chapter is to provide an introduction to the understanding of hypnosis within the context of pain management, especially focusing on clinical techniques relevant to the control of pain.

THE NATURE OF HYPNOSIS: AN OVERVIEW

The popular notion that hypnosis is a form of suggestibility is certainly an oversimplification (Hammer, Evans & Bartlett, 1963; Hilgard, 1965), even though this definition has dominated the otherwise impressive research on hypnotic phenomena from the 1930s (Hull, 1933), through the 1950s, (Weitzenhoffer, 1953) until now. Although it is agreed that response to suggestion is an important aspect of what happens during hypnosis, it is also generally agreed that hypnosis is a more complex phenomenon (Lynn & Rhue, 1991).

Some authors emphasize the social-psychological or social-cognitive interaction between the hypnotist and the subject as central to hypnotic behavior (Barber, 1969; Chaves & Brown, 1978; Diamond, 1977; Sarbin & Coe, 1972; Spanos, 1986; Wagstaff, 1981). For these authors, pain reduction involves interpersonal processes or self-generated cognitive and motivational strategies such as anxiety reduction, attribution, conditioning, distraction, focusing attention, forgetting, imagery, reallocation of attention away from the symptom, reframing, role playing, social contagion and compliance, and verbal relabeling. All of these strategies may be useful in controlling pain, especially when the pain is acute. In the social-psychological model, these strategies are facilitated by the hypnotic relationship, although it is often not clear how this is achieved. The hypnotic induction procedure itself and individual differences in hypnotic ability are usually considered incidental and unimportant.

Another view of hypnosis is that it reflects a stable capacity of the individual. It is viewed, often controversially, as a special state of consciousness, or, in psychodynamic theory, as a manifestation of the unconscious mind (Brown & Fromm, 1986). Some clinicians view hypnosis as the preferred way to access unconscious processes. Hypnosis may facilitate wishes or emotions, memories of trauma, and loosen defenses, mostly through the use of metaphor and guided imagery (Erickson, 1980; Rossi, 1993; Cheek, 1994). Such concepts are very difficult to test empirically, even though they may lead to compelling and clever clinical applications.

In a formulation that leads to more direct empirical investigation, hypnosis is considered in terms of dissociation theory. The hypnotic experience may involve an ability to readily change states of awareness or levels of consciousness. These changes in consciousness may be either interpersonally- or self-induced (Bowers, 1976; Evans, 1987; Hilgard, 1965, 1977). Hypnosis may be considered in terms of neodissociation theory or multiple cognitive pathways. For example, the pain patient simultaneously knows and does not know the severity of the pain. The awareness of pain and the analgesic experience are co-conscious (Hilgard, 1977). A similar process occurs during dental analgesia: during drilling, the patient reports feeling no pain, but retains the ability to know when the dentist is drilling at a site which should be painful, and even to know how much the drilling would hurt without the injection. In hypnosis, as in this example from dental analgesia, cognitive and somatic mechanisms are available to block or transform pain messages and sensations through controls in levels of consciousness. Pain awareness and hypnotic analgesia are co-conscious (Hilgard, 1977). Hypnosis may involve a more general cognitive flexibility, or switching mechanism, that allows one to change and control psychological, cognitive, or physiological processes, or readily access different levels of consciousness (Evans, 1987; 1991).

FOUR DIMENSIONS OF HYPNOTIC BEHAVIOR

It is useful to consider the domain of hypnosis as consisting of at least four conceptually independent constructs or dimensions. Noting which dimension an author is discussing will help the reader understand why hypnosis is a controversial field. Each dimension will have direct implications for the different ways hypnosis is practiced in the area of pain. Although these conceptual dimensions comprise the domain of hypnosis (Hilgard, 1973), most accounts of hypnosis usually focus on only one or two of them, leading to incomplete and even misleading conclusions.

1. *Expectations and Beliefs about Hypnosis*

The first of the four dimensions of hypnosis is an *expectation*, faith, or belief variable. It is probably common to any therapeutic modality and has its foundation in the special doctor-patient relationship. Laymen generally think of hypnosis as a quasi-magical technique, and also as something that is done to them. The typical chronic pain patient will arrive at a hypnosis treatment session with the expectation, "Doc, I understand that you're a hypnotist. Do it to me, fix me so I will feel better."

To appreciate the importance of expectations about hypnosis, note how much the practice of hypnosis has changed over the past 200 years. Considered the father of modern hypnosis, Mesmer is claimed to have hypnotized people by the thousands in Paris after he had been banished by the conservative Vienna medical establishment. The principles of physical magnetism had just been discovered. Mesmer (1779) argued that *animal magnetism,* or field forces that could be rearranged with magnets, could cure physical illness. At the height of his popular practice, he would hold seances where people would gather around tubs filled with water and iron filings, with metal rods protruding. When a participant arrived to be healed he or she would hold a metal rod, or hold somebody's hand, who in turn held a metal rod. As doctors do these days, Mesmer often arrived late (he often entertained ladies at the French Court), dressed in the purple robes of royalty (as some famous hypnotists still do, superstitiously). As many healers have done throughout the centuries, he would lay his hands on the nearest person. First that person, then the next person, as in a ripple effect through an audience, would immediately go into "hypnosis." What was hypnosis like then? One after the other, the participants fell to the ground and had a hysterical seizure. After the seizure, they fell into a deep sleep for a few seconds or sometimes several hours. When they awakened, they were allegedly cured of whatever ailed them. I personally know hundreds of colleagues who practice hypnosis with thousands of clients, but I do not know a single colleague who has reported that a patient went into trance, falling onto the floor with a seizure. In just 200 years, the nature of the hypnotic phenomenon has changed that much. This kind of behavioral compliance is not hypnosis. Responses may occur during a hypnotic session which may have nothing to do with hypnosis per se. They may be a result of the demands of the shared expectations and the need to be a compliant subject.

We (Evans & Mitchell, 1977) have shown this contagion-like compliance in hypnotic performance. During the administration of the

Harvard Group Scale of Hypnotic Susceptibility (HGSHS:A, Shor & Orne, 1962), subjects who sit next to each other score more alike than neighboring subjects sitting further apart. When the same subject pairs are compared on the individually administered Stanford Hypnotic Susceptibility Scale: Form C (SHSS:C, Weitzenhoffer & Hilgard, 1962), they no longer score more alike than previously non-neighboring subjects.

Hypnosis experienced a major resurgence in interest at the end of the nineteenth century when Bernheim (1889) introduced the now common view that hypnosis was merely a form of suggestion. It is still widely assumed that suggestibility increases during hypnosis, but this assumption has not been easy to document. It has been usually assumed that people are not suggestible in the normal waking state, and therefore, any response to suggestion during hypnosis must be due to hypnosis. This is like being surprised that a person who has red hair during hypnosis still has red hair when no longer in hypnosis (Hammer, Evans & Bartlett, 1963).

In conflict with Bernheim's suggestion theory, Charcot (1886) argued that hypnosis was a psychopathological phenomenon and was a form of hysteria. Charcot argued that only (hysterical) women could be hypnotized, although no sex differences in hypnotic ability have been consistently documented (Hilgard, 1965).

Freud was familiar with Charcot's observations and, influenced by his studies with Breuer on the abreactive cure (Breuer & Freud, 1924), his early work with hypnosis was instrumental in developing his theory of unconscious motivation (Ellenberger, 1970). Freud was later to give up hypnosis, giving as a reason that he could not hypnotize all of his patients. This is a surprising rationale: he never considered giving up free association or dream analysis because he couldn't make all patients associate freely or recall dreams. Freud's decision to discontinue using hypnosis highlights the crux of the lay person's view of hypnosis that the (malevolent) hypnotist controls the (gullible) patient's behavior (for suspicious motives). The lay person's view of hypnosis has been forged by two works of fiction—*Mario and the Magician* (Mann, 1930) and *Trilby* (Du Maurier, 1890)—in which hypnotists are depicted as irresistible exploiters of the innocent.

Most patients still think of hypnosis as a somewhat mysterious and magical technique in which they will be controlled by the hypnotist's suggestions, and they expect that they will have to accept uncritically whatever the hypnotist suggests. In an introductory lecture or seminar in hypnosis, I will often begin with a demonstration I learned from Martin Orne (personal communication). I ask the group if they will help me by loaning me a few objects. I walk around the room casually asking one participant if I can borrow his or her watch. I then ask another participant for her or his glasses. Next, I might ask a woman if I could have a piece of her jewelry (a necklace or a ring). I have usually caught the group's attention by the time I ask one of the men, "Could I have your wallet?" As I carry their valuable personal possessions back to the front of the room, I casually ask: "By the way, are any of the four of you hypnotized right now?" Invariably, with some bemusement, they say, "No." Then I point out to the group that if I had begun this demonstration by reciting a hypnotic induction ritual suggesting that they are relaxed and sleepy, etc., everybody present would have been convinced that hypnosis controlled the behavior of these four individuals! I was able to persuade them to give me their valuable possessions without hypnosis. My power to influence them was a function of the social context in which I obtained their possessions. Trust, the assumption that these requests had a purpose related to the course, or some other demand characteristic (Orne, 1959) of the safe situation, facilitated their compliance with my puzzling requests.

This powerful demonstration is convincing that social control and hypnosis are unrelated. Whatever hypnosis may be, it is not a method of increasing social control in the doctor-patient relationship. In fact, a goal of the therapist is to teach the patient that hypnosis may be the most powerful way to learn and increase self-control. Most contemporary practitioners of hypnosis reject the "control" issue and point out that all hypnosis is really self-hypnosis. The contemporary view of hypnosis is that the therapist's role is that of a teacher, guide, or mentor.

When I was a graduate student in the early 1960s, we typically took thirty minutes or more verbalizing hypnotic induction techniques. Even over the period of time that I have been working with hypnosis, its nature has changed dramatically. Now, patients take five minutes, or even thirty seconds, to go into hypnosis. Many therapists will tell you that you don't need an induction technique (Barber, 1977; Spiegel, 1970). Hypnosis has had a chameleon-like character over time! How can this be understood? We can't even describe the phenomenon that we're talking about because it often takes a form that the subject expects and, particularly, that the therapist expects.

What is considered an invariant characteristic of hypnosis by one investigator is considered an artifact by another. Contradictory markers of trance are vehemently espoused by clinicians, each of whom is convinced by his or her own beliefs about hypnosis. It can be found in the literature, for example, that the hypnotized person has a sense of humor, or has no sense of humor; has a fixed glassy stare, or has slow, or fast, or rolling eye movements; swallows frequently or hardly ever swallows; has or has not had spontaneous catalepsy; or amnesia, and so on. There is no scientific evidence to support any of these claims. Yet, each observation has validity in the sense that the behaviors are gradually shaped, and become part of the repertoire of the learned behaviors occurring during hypnotic interactions. Orne (1959) demonstrated a brand new criterion of hypnosis–catalepsy of the nondominant hand–but only in those subjects who watched a demonstration of hypnosis including the testing of this effect, without any verbal mention of its occurrence. It was never observed in subjects who watched a similar hypnosis demonstration, but without the testing of the "planted" nondominant catalepsy suggestion.

When one has an opportunity to watch a therapist demonstrate hypnosis, it is interesting to focus occasionally on the behavior of the hypnotist, not only the patient. The hypnotist's behavior often changes more dramatically than the patient's does, and certainly more than it does when he or she is doing any other form of therapy. Changes in posture, soft slower voice, attending to the patient's breathing closely, the strong but subtle changes in body language of both therapist and patient all contribute to the dramatic changes in beliefs and expectations of patient and therapist during hypnosis. These changes may have a powerful therapeutic influence! I like to refer to these firmly entrenched but undocumented beliefs about hypnosis as the hypnotist's/therapist's *superstitious behavior*. The therapist's influential superstitious behavior when using hypnosis will be molded largely by which of the four dimensions of hypnotic behavior the therapist considers most important.

The common expectational factors of all healing processes are best viewed as similar to the placebo or nonspecific effects that any technique will have (Frank, 1961; Evans, 1985). The placebo response is about 60 percent the magnitude of the treatment variable that is being investigated (Evans, 1981a, 1981c). The placebo response is about 60 percent as effective as morphine; it is about 60 percent as effective as aspirin; it is about 60 percent as effective as sleeping pills; and it is about 60 percent as effective as antidepressants (Evans, 1985). In other words, the effect of taking a pill, or the process of doing therapy, has something to do with the rituals of the therapeutic relationship and the expectations of getting well. When we believe that a treatment is powerful, we get powerful treatment results. The context in which any treatment modality is used makes an important contribution to therapeutic change. This holds for drugs, surgery, acupuncture, biofeedback, vitamin and herbal supplements, magnets, grandmother's favorite potion, and, of course, hypnosis. The label "hypnosis" evokes powerful expectations of change and therapeutic involvement which may be quite independent and possibly unrelated to the changes produced by the essential core of the hypnotic condition, whatever that is. This is the same mechanism as the placebo effect and it has powerful but independent effects compared to the drug the patient believes he or she is taking or the treatment being tried (Evans, 1991). The expectational or placebo effects of a treatment cannot be isolated easily from specific (e.g., hypnotic) treatment effects; yet failure to acknowledge these powerful but independent effects leads to much clinical confusion.

2. Suggestion and Hypnosis

The second important dimension of hypnosis is *suggestion*. Everybody knows that hypnosis has something to do with suggestion, but it is not clear what this term means (Hull, 1993; Weitzenhoffer, 1957; Evans, 1967). No objective laboratory measure of suggestion (whether it is of verbal suggestions of the body swaying backwards or forwards, of gullibility, of social conformity, of the contagion effect of crowds, of selling ice boxes to Eskimos) correlates very well with accepted hypnosis measurement scales. And yet whenever we use hypnosis, we are giving suggestions. That is a paradox! What do we mean by *suggestion*?

A group of subjects may be given suggestions for two minutes that "your arm is getting lighter and lighter, and it is floating up into the air, light as a balloon. Isn't it fascinating how easily it floats up into the air..." In about 80 percent of the subjects, the arm will float up into the air, some faster than others. For some, the arm will be nearly straight up; for some it will be just off the armrest. Only a few people will not have moved their arm at all. A much more effective way to have everybody raise his or her arm straight up would be the direct request: "Please everybody, raise your hand up in the air." This request would get a 100 percent response, instantaneously!

What is it that is so fascinating about taking two minutes to get some people to respond to suggestions by raising their arms, some to respond partially, and some not to respond at all? It is fascinating because of the subjective experience that accompanies the experience of the arm floating up. The suggestion implies that something *different* is going to happen. The arm has a "life of its own." Even though you could stop it anytime you wanted to, you wouldn't want to stop it, or perhaps you felt you couldn't stop it at all.

During hypnotic suggestions there is always a monitoring process going on, even though it sometimes seems very remote from conscious awareness. We become engaged in what the mind seems to be doing to a part of the body. The process of responding to suggestion engages our attention precisely because the arm seems to be floating nonvoluntarily or out of conscious control. We focus, we usually relax, and we are intrigued by this experience of responding to suggestions. In short, the suggestion involves not just the behavioral response as such but also the individual's subjective experience of the lifting. The observer would have to depend on the patient's report of what it was like, and his or her subjective experience. The report may or may not be congruent with what was observed.

In a group situation, there would be many unique experiences following that simple suggestion. The individual subject's report of differences in *how* one had that experience, not just that it happened, would be different for each person. The uniqueness of the experience is a key to the "stuff" of hypnotic behavior. For some in the group, the arm would not move in response to the suggestions. Some members of the group may have raised the arm because they expected it should happen, or because their neighbor responded (expectational component). Some may have focused on a balloon pulling up the arm (cognitive component). Others may have found the experience as surprising and/or out of conscious control (dissociative component). The clinician must pay close attention to the patient's report of his or her subjective experience, and the report may or may not be congruent with the therapist's observations. A variation of this simple direct suggestion is presented later and it is valuable as a first experience of responding to suggestion in a clinical population such as pain patients or patients with medical conditions.

Suggestion is an important component in treating pain with hypnosis. For example, simple suggestions can be given that the patient's hand is numb, and he or she can't feel anything. It might then be possible to transfer that numbness to the head (if the patient has a headache), and that the suggested anesthesia will take away the headache. This may be accompanied by the subjective experience that something interesting has happened to the hand and eventually perhaps to the headache. Sometimes suggestion can be augmented by naturally occurring subtle physiological reactions that are usually outside of the awareness of the subject. For example, glove analgesia can be facilitated by the therapist holding the subject's hand by the wrist, slightly occluding the pulse, thus creating some tingling leading to increased numbness in the hand. This can also be done by allowing the hand to rest over a sharp edge of the arm of the chair. Eye fixation leads readily to eye heaviness and the desire to close the eyes. If subtle suggestions are given to naturally occurring perceptual effects of eye fixation (blurring or movement of the fixation spot, tiredness, etc.), the eye closure is usually facilitated as the patient accepts the positive response as being due to the suggestion. Early reinforcement of such successful suggestions helps develop the expectation that each successful experience naturally leads to the success of the next suggestion (especially when it is left to the patient to help define what constitutes a successful response).

3. The Cognitive Dimension—Relaxation, Imagery and Trance Logic

The third dimension related to hypnosis is what might be broadly called a *cognitive* dimension. It has something to do with relaxation, with imagery, and with the distortions of perception, memory, cognition, and physiology that some have argued is the essence of hypnosis (Orne, 1959). The use of hypnosis to produce increased relaxation and imagery, positive and negative hallucinations, and perhaps age regression and analgesia are all described extensively in any text on hypnosis (Clarke & Jackson, 1983; Crasilneck & Hall, 1985; Hammond, 1990; Hunter 1994; Weitzenhoffer, 1957).

RELAXATION. Most hypnotic induction techniques focus on and even begin with procedures to facilitate deep physical and mental relaxation (Edmonston, 1981). For many patients, particularly those of low hypnotic ability, a hypnotic induction may not involve any more than the capacity for, and results obtained with, deep physical relaxation. However, the evidence seems to suggest that for at least some patients (usually those with higher hypnotic ability), hypnosis is somehow different from a variety of relaxation techniques, such as those based on Benson's (1975) brief relaxation response, the longer, deeper Jacobson (1938) progressive relaxation methods, or the myriad of available relaxation techniques that fall between these extremes.

Probably the most compelling evidence that hypnosis and relaxation differ stems from the work of Banyai and Hilgard (1976) and Vingoe (1968). For example, Banyai and Hilgard were able to show that deep hypnosis could be induced successfully while the subject was riding an exercise cycle. This technique is not especially relaxing for most subjects! Vingoe and others have also published about so-called active alert hypnosis, although most hypnotic induction techniques initially build on relaxation techniques.

The notion that the deeply hypnotized person is in an almost cataleptic-like or sleep-like state is part of what I call the superstitious behavior that is a legacy of the common lay notions of hypnosis in which trance is viewed as having something to do with sleep. The evidence shows that hypnosis and sleep produce different EEG patterns (Evans, 1979, 1981b, 1982; Crawford, 1990). Hypnosis produces an alert waking EEG, not one resembling sleep. Different relaxation techniques also differ from both hypnosis and sleep in their EEG patterns, some being associated with increased alpha, beta, theta, or even delta waves, which are characteristics not shared by the hypnosis EEG. There is consistent research, reviewed by Crawford (1990), showing that there are some differences in right and left hemisphere activation in hypnosis, but it is difficult to interpret the relative direction of the differences in activation in the two hemispheres.

IMAGERY. Imagery is a cornerstone of behavioral and psychological treatment techniques whether it is used with hypnosis or as a technique on its own. Imagery is an important component of hypnosis. Imagery is used creatively by the Ericksonian school whose adherents have mastered the art of guided imagery and metaphor as hypnotic techniques, often to access unconscious levels of awareness (Erickson, 1960; Rossi,1993).

There is still no clear evidence that imagery ability is increased by hypnosis, although it probably is. The vividness of imagery is far less important clinically than the ability to voluntarily manipulate and control the image. For example, I will use a suggestion that the patient is imagining lying on a peaceful beach. I enquire about his or her subjective experience for visual, auditory, olfactory, and somatic imagery ("can you see the waves?... hear the birds?... can you smell the fresh salt air?... feel the coolness of the breeze as the sun passes briefly behind a cloud?..."). I will then give a suggestion like, "Can you see a dog running along the beach?" When the patient responds "Yes," I ask "What color is it?" For example, if the patient responds "It is a brown dog," I ask whether he or she can "see it as not a brown dog, I think it is really another color." If the image is static, like an image on a TV screen, and the patient does not seem able to change the channel, this imagery is not very useful in clinical practice. It is the patient who can control or flexibly change the image immediately, and who can make the color change, who provides the basis for solid utilization of imagery in hypnosis. One of the earliest suggestions I will use with pain patients is to ask him or her, "What color is your pain?" Typically the response is red or black. I then ask, "What is your favorite color." I will explore ways in which the patient can scan the redness (or color of the pain) and gradually change it into a soothing, calm green (or whatever is the favorite color).

An even more critical point about imagery and hypnosis is the frequent but erroneous assumption that imagery is primarily visual. Indeed, chronic pain patients often do not have good flexible visual imagery, but have good imagery in other modalities, particularly sensory, kinesthetic, and somatic. For example, a suggestion of "feeling the muscle tissue being as soft and smooth as satin or silk," or changing "the muscles from the coarse, hard, brittle, breakable, cold feeling of uncooked spaghetti into the soft, squiggly, loose, smooth, warm feeling of cooked spaghetti" is often more useful to pain patients than cleverly constructed visually-oriented guided imagery.

TRANCE LOGIC. One of the defining characteristics of hypnosis is the ability of the deeply hypnotized subject to experience what Orne (1959, 1974) has called "trance logic." The hypnotized patient is readily able to tolerate logical inconsistencies in perception, cognition, physiology, and sensation. For example, a deeply hypnotized subject, when asked to forget all about the number "6," and then when asked to count his or her fingers, will be puzzled, but not too distressed, to discover he or she has an extra eleventh digit. Using a complex and special methodology that asks unhypnotizable subjects to fake hypnosis to a blind experimenter (Orne, 1959), the simulating subject will find clever ways to not use the number "6" when counting his or her fingers but will nevertheless avoid coming up with the solution of an eleventh digit! For example, a subject might count "1, 2, 3, 4, 5, and 5 more is 10," while displaying the five digits on the other hand (Evans, 1974). The ability to tolerate logical inconsistencies is one of the best documented characteristics of hypnosis, and is only found with highly hypnotizable subjects. Trance logic may relate to dissociative experiences of hypnosis and the "hidden observer" technique described by Hilgard (1977) for studying hypnotic analgesia.

POSITIVE AND NEGATIVE HALLUCINATIONS. The judicious use of positive and negative hallucinations with the pain patient will facilitate pain management. For example, I might suggest that a patient with chronic back pain will learn how to hallucinate a pain in his or her shoulder and then give suggestions of removing that pain. This sends a message to the patient that at least in some sense, pain control is possible and may well be transferred later to the pain in the back. Suggestion of warmth or cold in a limb that is not a pain site may have a similar use. A suggestion of hand or glove analgesia can often be transferred to the site of the real pain to reduce the suffering.

4. The Dissociation Component of Hypnosis

The fourth component of hypnosis is dissociation. It is probably the core of what is usually considered deep hypnosis. It is the basis of some of the more dramatic hypnotic phenomena including posthypnotic amnesia, posthypnotic suggestion, negative hallucinations, age regression, anesthesia, and analgesia. Dissociation has something to do with being able to focus attention, and to attend selectively to stimuli, or to block them out of awareness. For example, most of us have had the experience of getting caught up or absorbed in a good book, or losing track of time. Somebody might come into the room and speak to the reader who is too absorbed to notice the visitor for awhile; but then suddenly "knows" the appropriate response. Many people can cry at a sad movie, getting absorbed and identifying with the action, being able to put external reality aside temporarily. Most have had the experience of driving home after a long day, trying to solve a problem, and all of sudden realizing, "I'm home—I don't remember that dangerous traffic circle (or busy intersection)." However, if there had been a "near miss," attention would have been reallocated instantaneously from "automatic pilot" to careful navigation through the circle at the temporary expense of the problem solving.

A good illustration of dissociation is the following question: "Have you have fallen out of bed recently?" Almost everybody answers "no," with a smile. Typically, we move about the bed several times every night with gross body movements. Nevertheless, we are able to monitor the edge of the bed so that we never fall out. Children need to learn this. Not only do we monitor the edge of the bed, we monitor our sleeping partner's position—if one moves to the wrong side of the bed, one gets a good swift kick, but neither partner wakes up! If you have a baby in the next room and it starts to cry faintly, you immediately wake up—the so-called *mother-cry* phenomenon. Yet a loud fire engine will go by, but it is not even heard. We are automatically monitoring our environment totally out of awareness, at a complex level all the time.

A body of research has shown that subjects with high hypnotic ability perform better on activities that seem to depend on normal everyday dissociative skills (Bowers, 1985; Evans, 1991; Hilgard, 1977). It seems that dissociation may be a normal individual difference dimension, of which hypnotic capacity is a key defining variable. It is well documented that highly hypnotizable subjects become more easily absorbed in daily experiences (Shor, 1960; Tellegen & Atkinson, 1976). People who are more hypnotizable are more likely to arrive late occasionally for appointments. They get caught up in what they are doing, and time slips by. Sometimes they turn up for appointments on the wrong day (Markowsky & Evans, 1978). People who are highly hypnotizable fall asleep more easily at night, apparently because they can switch easily between different states of consciousness (Evans, 1981b, 1989, 1991). They are more likely to be nappers and they nap to make up for lost sleep whenever they have the opportunity, or even when not tired (Evans, 1989, 1991). There is a flexibility of slipping in and out of dissociated states, whether it is sleep, hypnosis, and probably other states of consciousness that can be developed into techniques to control bodily functions including pain.

We have studied psychiatric patients with various diagnoses, unselected for hypnotic ability, and with whom hypnosis has not been used in treatment during their therapy. Highly hypnotizable psychiatric patients who have the capacity to experience hypnosis showed more improvement clinically within three months of hospitalization, even though hypnosis was not used in the therapy, compared to less hypnotizable patients. Two years later, however, the hypnotizable patients are more likely to be rehospitalized (Horne, Evans & Orne, 1983; Evans, 1989, 1991). Dissociation may be a double-edged sword. It may produce symptoms as well as being a positive factor leading to symptomatic improvement.

The nature of dissociation is illustrated by an old case study reported by Bagby (1928). Bagby relates the case of a teenage girl he was unsuccessfully treating for phobia of running water. One day the girl reported that an aunt, whom she had not seen since she was four years old, had come to town and had greeted her with this statement: "I have never told, have you?" The aunt subsequently confirmed that when she was babysitting for the four-year-old girl, she had fallen asleep in the park. The little girl had wandered off to play in a small waterfall. Her screams of terror awakened the aunt, who, because of her own guilt, threatened the girl to secrecy. Not surprisingly, hypnotic age regression and abreaction techniques, in which the girl reexperienced the trauma psychologically by being placed back under the waterfall so that she could discover that she had been removed safely from it, led to a dramatic cure.

Such case reports involving the acquisition of symptoms under stress-induced dissociative experiences are common, although it is rare that there is documentation of the occurrence of the stressful circumstance. This view of dissociation has more in common with the clinical literature on posttraumatic stress syndrome (which is often relevant to chronic pain produced by trauma such as motor vehicle and other accidents). This concept of dissociation is less related to the current surge in interest in so-called multiple personality, which may be related in complex ways to expectations (of the therapist as well as the patient) as well as shades of meaning of the term "dissociation."

My hypothesis is that there are significant individual differences in a dimension of personality and/or cognitive functioning that has something to do with the degree of control with which people can access different states of consciousness, psychological awareness, physiological change, or cognitive functioning (Evans, 1991; Bowers, 1985). Recognizing that there are many different usages of the term, I choose to label this individual-difference dimension "dissociation." Several converging lines of evidence suggest that the individual differences in the ability to experience hypnosis may reflect one aspect of a more general ability to access, regulate, and alter states of consciousness.

In the water phobia case described above, running water served as a *trigger,* which stimulated some form of reverbatory neural circuit representing a part of the little girl's psyche that was still panicking under the waterfall. This memory trace was dissociated. The hyper-aroused panic state was activated unconsciously by any stimulus that reminded her of running water. At some level she was still trapped under the waterfall. This (dissociated) panic was retriggered by any stimulus associated with running water. I would hypothesize that chronic pain may be triggered at times by a similar "loop" related to associations with the onset of the pain. The triggering stimuli may have little or no correlation with the anatomical structures where the patient localizes the (chronic) pain. Pain may involve a repetitive communication loop between a dissociated short circuiting area of the brain and the neural circuits communicating with the site of the pain. Chronic pain may involve faulty communication within the mind body system more than a localized peripheral site where the pain is experienced.

The ability to experience hypnosis may involve an important psychological dimension concerned with the control of consciousness. This dimension of labile accessibility to multiple levels of awareness has significant implications for understanding a wide range of psychological and physiological phenomena, some of which may have clinical significance concerning the development and alleviation of symptoms.

THE MEASUREMENT OF HYPNOSIS

It is generally agreed that there are important individual differences in the ability to experience hypnosis. Most existing scales to measure hypnotic susceptibility present a series of graded suggestions which sample the consensus domain of hypnosis. These suggestions are usually administered in a verbatim standardized manner. There are objective criteria to determine whether the subject has passed or failed a suggestion. The subject's score is the number of suggestions passed using an arbitrarily defined criterion. An important assumption is that the observed behavioral response to a suggestion reflects the subjective experience of the person completing the suggestion. It has been shown that the agreement between the subjective response of the subject and the observed response of the tester is extremely high (O'Connell, 1964; Weitzenhoffer & Hilgard, 1959, 1962).

It is important to note that the better hypnotic susceptibility scales such as the Stanford Hypnotic Susceptibility Scales (SHSS:A; SHSS:C) of Weitzenhoffer and Hilgard (1959, 1962), the Harvard Group Scale of Hypnotic Susceptibility (HGSHS:A) of Shor and Orne (1962), and the Hypnotic Induction Profile (HIP) of Spiegel and Bridger (1970) have psychometric and standardization properties of reliability and validity that are at least the equal of accepted individual ability and intelligence tests. As with the intelligence tests, there is room to debate what the scales measure. Research has shown that the retest reliability of SHSS:C is high (about .8) even after a 30-year retest period (Morgan & Hilgard, 1974).

Most research suggests that hypnotic ability cannot be modified in experimental settings. However, the frequent clinical assumption that hypnotic susceptibility may increase under highly motivated clinical conditions has not been tested. Motivation may well increase behavioral compliance and expectations rather than hypnotic ability itself. Some of the problems involved in the measurement of hypnosis in the clinic have been addressed thoroughly by Frankel (1976). If there are individual differences in hypnotizability (Hilgard, 1965), it is clearly inadequate to define hypnosis in terms of an induction procedure (Hull, 1933; Barber, 1969; Spanos, 1986). Screening for hypnotizability must be done carefully in clinical studies, including those about hypnotic pain control. Many studies do not carefully select extreme high and low hypnotizable subjects (Frankel, 1976). If hypnosis involves a unique set of skills, then subjects who have been selected for high hypnotizability will have the best opportunity to experience phenomena such as hypnotic analgesia and anesthesia.

It is difficult to get stable measures of hypnotizability without using two or three scales such as the SHSS:A, SHSS:C (Weitzenhoffer & Hilgard, 1959, 1962), the HIP (Spiegel & Spiegel, 1978), and the HGSHS:A (Shor & Orne, 1962). The initial hypnosis session tends to be contaminated by preconceptions, curiosities, and anxieties about the meaning of hypnosis. This is even more complicated in the clinic because a hypnotized patient may respond well to hypnosis during a screening session, but may refuse to experience hypnosis in a subsequent therapeutic context because of an unreadiness to give up the symptom, such as pain, and other forms of resistance. Therefore, it is critically important to evaluate hypnotic ability in the clinic independently of the treatment session so that hypnotic ability will not be confounded by the desire to be helpful or the impact of an unreadiness to get better.

THE INDUCTION OF HYPNOSIS

There are a number of excellent discussions of the induction and utilization of hypnosis (Clark & Jackson, 1983; Crasilneck & Hall, 1985; Erickson,1980; Hammond, 1990; Hunter,1994; Weitzenhoffer, 1957). These and other sources present verbatim scripts covering many hypnotic inductions and suggestions, from the standard to the very creative, and scripts for suggestions in almost every conceivable clinical application, symptom, or condition. Such inductions and scripts will not be presented here. The newcomer to the field should consider attending workshops introducing hypnosis (usually lasting 20 or more hours) sponsored by one of the professional hypnosis societies. Participation in the courses taught or sponsored by the International Society of Hypnosis, and national organizations such as the American Society of Clinical Hypnosis and The Society of Clinical and Experimental Hypnosis, and equivalent Societies in many other countries, is recommended. All such professional organizations limit training to health professionals with terminal degrees and national licensure (usually in *MEDICINE, DENTISTRY, PSYCHOLOGY, SOCIAL WORK AND NURSING*).

There is no "best" induction technique. It is the melody rather than the lyrics that lead to successful work with hypnosis. Hypnosis should be a comfortable fit between the style of the therapist and the unique needs of the patient. It is safe for a therapist to consider using hypnosis only when he or she knows that he or she would be competent to treat the patient's current problem even if he or she was not familiar with hypnosis.

This section will present three useful brief hypnotic techniques that are especially helpful during the early sessions with patients. The aim of these suggestions is to teach the person what it means to respond to suggestion, to let him or her experience the mind body influence that is so important to pain management, and to teach a very rapid technique for entering (self) hypnosis. These techniques provide a first step to help engender expectations that similar techniques of mind body control might help to control pain. These techniques are brief, novel, and are usually found to be surprisingly effective by the patient.

1. Differential Arm Levitation Technique

I usually use this as the first experience the patient will have with responding to suggestions. Depending on the circumstances, the therapist may or may not label this as an hypnotic procedure.

The suggestion should be administered in a soft, slow tone of voice. It should take two and a half to three minutes to administer. It need not be verbatim. Use suggestive voice intonation: the voice falls during "heaviness" suggestion, rises during the "lightness" suggestion.

We will now do a simple procedure to give you an opportunity to feel what it is like to respond to a suggestion. It will help if you close your eyes, and let yourself breathe a little slower and deeper than usual.

Pause 20 Seconds

Good. Now please hold both of your hands straight out, palms facing upwards. That's right, just a little higher.

(Demonstrate by adjusting the arms' positions so they are straight and slightly above the horizontal position. With the following suggestions, words _underlined_ should be emphasized, with voice modulation consistent with the suggested response and preferably in rhythm with the subject's exhalation.)

I want you to imagine what it would feel like if your _right_ arm begins to get _heavy_ . . . _heavier_ and _heavier_ . . . so _heavy_ you'll have difficulty in holding it up. Your arm will feel so _heavy_, so hard to hold up, that it will begin to fall _down_ . . . _down_ . . . _down_ . . . _heavier_ and _heavier_. . . . Good.

At the same time I want you to think of your _left_ arm _floating_ up into the air . . . feeling _lighter_ . . . and _lighter_ . . . and _lighter_. So _light_ . . . _way_ up into the air.

The right hand and arm feels _heavy_ . . . the left hand and arm feels _light_ . . . _floating_ up into the air. Right arm _heavier_ and _heavier_, and _heavier_. _Down_ . . . way _down_. . . . Good. The _left_ hand is feeling _lighter and lighter, and lighter_ . . . as if a balloon were pulling it up into the air. So _light_ . . . a large, pretty balloon. _Way up_ into the air. Right hand _heavier_, being pulled down by a _weight_. . . . Left hand so light it _floats_ way up into the air. . . . _Higher_, and _higher_, and _higher_.

Pause 10 Seconds

That's fine. Now just place both hands down in a comfortable position . . . and open your eyes.

Typically, 9 out of 10 patients will acknowledge a subjective response to this suggestion, although often it will only involve downward movement to the heaviness suggestion. I take the opportunity to point out that this is an example of how quite similar suggestions often produce different results, and that some suggestions are harder than others. This suggestion and its response may be the first acknowledgement by the patient that what one thinks about does influence what happens physically to the body. It is often a dramatic insight.

It is helpful to engage in some discussion with the patient to elicit comments about his/her subjective experience, and perceived differences in suggestion-difficulty between the arms. I usually inquire about how far apart the arms were at the end of the suggestion as patients often mis-estimate this. The subjective response is at least as important as the objective movement. I give the patient an opportunity to acknowledge that the suggestion seemed to work, although I have not given him or her any clue as to how far "up" and "down" constitutes a successful response. That is the patient's subjective interpretation.

Because most patients don't realize that holding the arm up for two to three minutes would produce some feelings of heaviness anyhow, it is likely that a patient who does not report a success with the heaviness suggestion is resisting at some level. If that is the case, other techniques would be introduced, such as the use of the Chevreul Pendulum, or a discussion of what the patient was thinking about during the procedure.

I will also inquire about whether the suggestion of the balloon pulling the left hand, and then a weight on the right hand, helped the response, thereby introducing the role of imagery as a facilitator of the experience. Some patients will already be using imagery before the balloon suggestion is given. A more hypnotizable patient may give a larger response to the lightness, rather than the heaviness, or occasionally will even hallucinate his or her arms moving even though no movement actually occurred. Although I do not mention this to the patient, notice how I reinforced the suggestion several times. I changed the suggestion from "your arm" to "the arm" to facilitate dissociative experiences.

Even a brief procedure like this provides a wealth of clinical information about the way the patient will respond to later suggestions and how mastery and body-mind self-control will be experienced.

2. The Eye Roll Relaxation Procedure

This is a transcript of a brief self-hypnosis procedure used in a number of clinical and medical settings. It is adapted from Herbert Spiegel, originally in the treatment of smoking (Spiegel, 1970). However it can be applied to almost any area of behavioral medicine and mind body healing. I present it as one of the quickest available methods of learning self-hypnosis, or as a psychological "time out" from whatever stressor is occurring at that moment. I sometimes teach it as a "short hypnosis" to be used when it is needed, and as an effective and rapid response to any stress. It can be a first step to enter a longer hypnotic trance, when there is more time and need to use it. This longer hypnosis will usually include techniques utilizing deep breathing, ego strengthening, relaxation, and future-oriented special place imagery.

The patient is asked to sit comfortably in the chair (without contact lenses if so desired).

I am going to teach you a very rapid way to learn self-hypnosis (or relaxation). The method requires you to do three things at once. It sounds more complex that it is, so first let me tell you what will happen, then I will do it for you as you watch, and only then will I ask you to try it.

The first thing is to take a very deep breath and hold it.

The second thing is to roll up your eyes to the very top of your head, and hold it.

The third thing is to hold your eyes in that position, and as you slowly close your eyelids, breathe out slowly, and relax.

Now, let me show you what happens. (The therapist repeats as above, demonstrating each step of the procedure.)

One, take a comfortable deep breath . . . and hold it.

Two, roll up your eyes as far as you can to the top of your head. . . . Good. . . . Three, as you hold your eyes in that position . . . slowly close your eyelids as you breathe out . . . and feel that wonderful wave of relaxation flow down through your body. . . .

That's great!

You can open your eyes. Now tell me what it felt like.

Repeat the procedure as reinforcement two or three times as necessary before an inquiry about the subjective experience is conducted.

I may rationalize this technique to the patient by indicating that the deep breath causes more oxygen exchange which facilitates biochemical reactions that result in feelings of physical relaxation. The eye movement procedure changes brain wave activity towards a more relaxed (alpha) mental state. The physical and mental relaxation produced by this procedure reinforces each other, so that it acts very quickly. Following Spiegel, I tell the patient *that this procedure can be used absolutely anywhere because it is so quick. It is so quick that it can be done even at a red traffic light.* I encourage the patient to use this technique to relax, and to reduce tension, for example, when feeling angry, or have other negative emotions welling up, and when pain is first increasing. I urge the patient to practice the technique at least 10 times a day for a week when not stressed or in severe pain, because the most difficult part of this method is to remember to use it when he or she needs it. When in the company of other people, the patient only needs to take a deep breath and blink, rather than rolling the eyes, perhaps emphasizing the tension reduction cycle by making a closed fist behind the back instead of using the eye roll. Following the procedure used by Spiegel and Spiegel (1978), a simple positive suggestion or affirmation can be used as the patient relaxes.

Although there is clinical lore suggesting that the amount of white during the eye roll technique predicts measured hypnotic ability, the actual correlation between the eye roll and measured hypnotizability is not very high (Orne, Hilgard, Spiegel, Spiegel, Crawford, Evans, Orne, & Stern, 1979). It should not by itself be used as a measure of hypnotic ability. Some clinicians inappropriately use a poor eye roll as an indication of low hypnotic ability, setting up unfortunate expectations that hypnosis may not be useful for this patient.

3. The Ideomotor Movement Response

This technique is directly derived from common sports medicine applications, especially for athletes in individual sports such as golf, figure skating, and gymnastics. However, I first learned it from Neal Miller (personal communication), who independently suggested it for controlling orthostatic hypotension. It is based on the principles of ideomotor action. This is an excellent technique to help improve movement in arthritic and joint pain, and those who find it very difficult to get up in the morning because of the stiffness and inability to get the body moving. It works when the patient has been lying down or sitting still for a long time as an aid to initiating movement.

I use the example of getting out of a chair, preferably after the patient has been sitting for 30–45 minutes. I invite the patient to get comfortable in the chair, relaxed with the eyes closed.

While you are relaxed, I want you think what it would feel like if you were actually getting up from the chair. Don't do it just yet. Just imagine <u>all</u> of the sensations that you would experience if you were <u>actually</u> getting up from the chair. . . . Perhaps you can <u>see</u> yourself getting up from the chair... or perhaps you can just <u>feel</u> the movements that your body would go through if you were actually getting up from the chair. <u>Scan</u> your body memories for what movements you might make if you were <u>getting up</u> from the chair. . . . Just visualize and imagine and feel this in any way that feels <u>comfortable</u> for you. Just spend a few moments working on imagining and experiencing what it would feel like if you were actually getting up from the chair.

Pause about 30 seconds

This suggestion might be reinforced for a short period of time, allowing a period of silence. It is not necessary to rehearse the imagery for more than 90 seconds to two minutes. I then ask the patient to open his or her eyes and then get up from the chair.

When the patient is seated again, he or she is likely to express pleasant surprise at how much easier it was to get out of the chair than normal after 45 minutes or so. I explain that this technique can be used when getting out of bed in the morning, or any other time tightness and stiffness is felt. I explain that this is a principle derived from sports psychology (Unesthal, 1976), where athletes use this kind of ideomotor imagery to rehearse their perfect performance. Imaging and visualizing the required performance is akin to "priming the pump" for the body. The body is actually remembering the movements of previous successful performance and becomes primed to replicate those movements in terms of subliminal proprioceptive cues, changes in peripheral blood flow, oxygen use, biochemical involvement, and nerve transmission. I point out that if the patient were trying to use this technique to improve their golf or tennis game, he or she can well imagine what would happen if the procedure were used to rehearse mistakes rather than perfect performance. Patients find the procedure to be intuitively appealing, and often continue to use it indefinitely. This technique is an excellent illustration of the use of ideomotor action imagery as a clinical technique for mind-body control. It is the basis of some later powerful techniques in the management of pain using self-control skills.

SUMMARY

This chapter has provided a short introduction to hypnosis. It is not intended to replace a more detailed discussion of hypnosis and its many clinical applications that can be found in many excellent treatments, some of which are listed in the references. Nor, for the newcomer to hypnosis, is it intended to substitute for an introductory course on hypnosis. The chapter provides a brief history of hypnosis, especially relevant to pain management. It then presents a conceptual framework to help the reader understand some controversies in the literature, and a means of understanding some important differences and disagreements in the field. It is this author's view that hypnotic responses can be understood as a complex mix of four conceptual (and empirical) dimensions: *expectations*, akin to the placebo response; *suggestion*; a *cognitive* component including relaxation, imagery in all modalities, and trance logic; *dissociation*, which is seen as the key component of deep hypnosis, and which may involve individual differences the flexible control of experience. There is a brief discussion of the importance of measuring individual differences in hypnotic ability using some of the better hypnosis measuring scales. Finally, three brief and useful innovative hypnotic techniques are described that are useful in the earlier sessions to introduce the pain patient to powerful mind-body interventions that can be used at any time by the suffering patient.

REFERENCES

Bagby, E. (1928). *The psychology of personality.* New York: Holt.
Banyai, E., & Hilgard, E.R. (1976). A comparison of active-alert hypnotic induction with traditional relaxation induction. *Journal of Abnormal Psychology, 85,* 218–224.
Barber, J. (1977). Rapid induction analgesia: A clinical report. *American Journal of Clinical Hypnosis, 19,* 138–147.
Barber, T.X. (1969). *Hypnosis: A scientific approach.* New York: Van Nostrand.
Bennet, Benson, & Kuiken. (1986). Preoperative instructions for decreased bleeding

during spinal surgery. *Anesthesiology, 63,* 245.

Benson, H. (1975). *The relaxation response.* New York: Morrow.

Bernheim, H. (1889: Trans. C.A. Herter). *Suggestive therapeutics: A treatise on the nature and uses of hypnotism.* New York: Putnam.

Bowers, K.S. (1985). *Hypnosis for the seriously curious.* New York: Norton.

Breuer, J., & Freud, S. (1924: Trans. J. Rickman). *Collected Papers,* Vol. 1. London: Hogarth.

Brown, D.E., & Fromm, E. (1986). *Hypnotherapy and hypnoanalysis.* Hilllsdale, NJ: Lawrence Erlbaum.

Charcot, J.M. (1886). *Oeuvres Completes du Progrès Médical,* Paris. 9 Vols.

Chaves, J.F., & Brown, J.M. (1978). *Self-generated strategies for the control of pain and stress.* Paper presented at the Annual Meeting of the American Psychological Association, Toronto, Canada.

Cheek, D.B. (1994). Hypnosis: *The application of ideomotor procedures.* Boston: Bacon.

Clarke, J.C., & Jackson, J.A. (1983). *Hypnosis and behavior therapy: The treatment of anxiety and phobias.* New York: Springer.

Crasilneck, H.B., & Hall, J.A. (1985). *Clinical hypnosis: Principles and applications.* New York: Grune and Stratton.

Crawford, H.J. (1990). Cognitive and psychophysiological correlates of hypnotic responsiveness and hypnosis. In M.L. Fass & D.P. Brown (Eds.), *Creative mastery in hypnosis and hypnoanalysis: A Festschrift for Erika Fromm* (pp. 155–168). Hillsdale, NJ: Lawrence Erlbaum.

Diamond, M.J. (1977). Hypnotizability is modifiable: An alternative approach. *International Journal of Clinical and Experimental Hypnosis, 25,* 147–165.

Domangue, B.B., & Margolis, C.G. (1983). Hypnosis and a multidisciplinary cancer pain management team: Role and effects. *International Journal of Clinical and Experimental Hypnosis, 31,* 206–212.

Dubin, L.L., & Shapiro, S. (1974). The use of hypnosis to facilitate a dental extraction and hemostasis in a classic hemophiliac with a high antibody titre to Factor 8. *American Journal of Clinical Hypnosis, 17,* 79–83.

DuMaurier, G. *(1890). Trilby.* New York, Dutton.

Edmonston, W.E. (1981). *Hypnosis and relaxation: Modern verification of an old equation.* New York: John Wiley.

Ellenberger, H.F. (1970). *The discovery of the unconscious: The history and evolution of psychiatry.* New York: Basic Books.

Erickson, M.H. Deep hypnosis and its induction. In L.E. LeCron (Ed.), *Experimental hypnosis.* New York: Macmillan.

Erickson, M.H. (1980). *The collected papers of Milton H. Erickson on hypnosis. Volumes 1–4.* Edited by E.L. Rossi, M.O.Ryan, & F.A. Sharp (Eds.), New York, Irvington.

Esdaile, J. (1957). *Hypnosis in medicine and surgery.* New York: Julian Press. (Originally entitled Mesmerism in India, 1850).

Evans, F.J. (1967). Suggestibility in the normal working state. *Psychological Bulletin, 67,* 114–129.

Evans, F.J. (1974, October). Sixes on the tip-of-the tongue: Problem solving during specific hypnotic amnesia. In A.M. Weitzenhoffer (Chair), *Suggested inability to recall.* Symposium presented at the 26th Annual Meeting of the Society of Clinical and Experimental Hypnosis, Montreal.

Evans, F.J. (1979). Hypnosis and sleep: Techniques for exploring cognitive activity during sleep. In E. Fromm & R.E. Shor (Eds.), *Hypnosis: Research developments and perspectives* (Rev. ed.). Chicago: Aldine.

Evans, F.J. (1981a). Hypnosis, placebo, and the control of pain. *Scandinavian Journal of Clinical and Experimental Hypnosis, 8,* 69–76.

Evans, F.J. (1981b). Sleep and hypnosis: Accessibility of altered states of consciousness. *Advanced Physiological Science, 17,* 453–456.

Evans, F.J. (1981c). The placebo response in pain control. *Psychopharmacological Bulletin, 17,* 72–76.

Evans, F.J. (1982). Hypnosis and sleep. Research Communications in Psychology, *Psychiatry and Behavior, 7,* 241–256.

Evans, F.J. (1985). Expectancy, therapeutic instructions, and the placebo response. In L. White, B.Tursky, & G. Schwartz, (Eds.), *Placebo: Clinical phenomena and new insights.* New York: Guilford Press.

Evans, F.J. (1987). Hypnosis and chronic pain. In G.D. Burrows, D. Elton, & R. Stanley, (Eds.), *Handbook of chronic pain management.* Amsterdam, Holland: Elsevier.

Evans, F.J. (1989). The hypnotizable patient. In D. Waxman, D. Pedersen, I. Wilkie, & P. Mellett (Eds.), *Hypnosis: The Fourth European Congress at Oxford* (pp. 18–28). London: Whurr.

Evans, F.J. (1991). Hypnotizability: Individual differences in dissociation and the flexible control of psychological processes. In S.J. Lynn & J.W. Rhue, (Eds.), *Theories of hypnosis.* New York: Guilford.

Evans, F.J. (in press, b.). Hypnosis in management of chronic pain. In L.E. Fredericks (Ed.), *The use of hypnosis in surgery and anesthesiology.* Springfield, Illinois, Charles C Thomas.

Evans, F.J., & Mitchell, W.A. (1977, October). Interaction between neighbors during hypnosis: The independence of social influence and hypnotizability. Paper presented at the 29th Scientific Meeting of the Society of Clinical and Experimental Hypnosis, Los Angeles.

Frank, J.D. (1972). *Persuasion and healing.* Baltimore: Johns Hopkins Press.

Frankel, F. H. (1976). *Trance as a coping mechanism.* New York: Plenum.

Hammer, A. G., Evans, F.J., & Bartlett, M. (1963). Factors in hypnosis and suggestion. *Journal of Abnormal and Social Psychology, 67,* 15–23.

Hammond, D.C. (Ed.). (1990). *Handbook of hypnotic suggestions and metaphors.* New York: Norton.

Hilgard, E.R. (1965). *Hypnotic susceptibility.* New York: Harcourt, Brace & World.

Hilgard, E.R. (1973). The domain of hypnosis, with some comments on alternative paradigms. *American Psychologist, 28,* 972–982.

Hilgard, E.R. (1977). *Divided consciousness: Multiple controls in human thought and action.* New York: John Wiley & Sons.

Hilgard, E.R., & Hilgard, J.R. (1975). *Hypnosis in the relief of pain.* Los Altos, CA:

William Kaufman, Inc.

Horne, R.L., Evans, F.J., & Orne, M.T. (1983, October). *Hypnotizability and treatment outcome in hospitalized psychiatric patients.* Paper presented at the annual meeting of the Society for Clinical and Experimental Hypnosis, Boston.

Hull, C.L. (1933). *Hypnosis and suggestibility: An experimental approach.* New York: Appleton-Century-Crofts.

Hunter, M.E. (1994). *Creative scripts for hypnotherapy.* New York: Brunner Mazel.

Jacobson, E. (1938). *Progressive relaxation.* Chicago: Chicago of University Press.

Lynn, S.J. & Rhue, J.W. *Theories of hypnosis.* New York: Guilford.

Mann, T. (1930). *Mario the Magician.* New York, Dutton.

Markowsky, P.A., & Evans, F.J. (1978, October*).* *Occasional lateness for appointments in hypnotizable subjects.* Paper presented at the 30th Annual Meeting of the Society for Clinical and Experimental Hypnosis, Asheville, NC.

Mesmer, F.A. (1779). *Mémoire sur la Découverté du Magnétisme Animal.* Geneva, Switzerland.

Morgan, A. H., Johnson, D.L., & Hilgard, E.R. (1974). The stability of hypnotic susceptibility: A longitudinal study. *International Journal of Clinical and Experimental Hypnosis, 22,* 245–257.

O'Connell, D.N. (1964). An experimental comparison of hypnotic depth measured by self-ratings and by an objective scale. *International Journal of Clinical and Experimental Hypnosis, 12,* 34–46.

Orne, M.T. (1959). The nature of hypnosis. Artifact and essence. *Journal of Abnormal Psychology, 46,* 213–225.

Orne, M.T. (1974). Pain suppression by hypnosis and related phenomena. In J.J. Bonica(Ed.), *Pain.* New York: Raven Press.

Orne, M.T., Hilgard, E.R., Spiegel, H., Spiegel, D., Crawford, H.J., Evans, F.J., Orne, E.C., & Stern, D.B. (1979). The Hypnotic Induction Profile as a measure of hypnotizability: Its internal characteristics and relation to the Stanford Hypnotic Susceptibility Scales, Forms A and C. *International Journal of Clinical and Experimental Hypnosis,* 27, 85–102.

Rossi, E.L. (1993). *The Psychobiology of Mind-Body Healing: New Concepts of Therapeutic Hypnosis.* New York: Norton.

Sacerdote, P. (1970). Theory and practice of pain control in malignancy and other protracted or recurring painful illnesses. *International Journal of Clinical and Experimental Hypnosis, 18, 160–180.*

Sarbin, T.R., & Coe, W. (1972). *Hypnosis: A Social Psychological Analysis of Influence Communication.* New York: Holt, Rinehart & Winston.

Shor, R.E. (1960). The frequency of naturally occurring "hypnotic-like" experiences in the normal college population. *International Journal of Clinical and Experimental Hypnosis, 8,* 151–163.

Shor, R.E., & Orne, E.C. (1962). *Harvard Group Scale of Hypnotic Susceptibility, Form A.* Palo Alto, CA: Consulting Psychologists Press.

Spanos, N.P. (1986). A social psychological approach to hypnotic behavior. *Behavior and Brain Sciences, 9,* 449–467.

Spiegel, H. (1970). A single-treatment method to stop smoking using ancillary self-hypnosis. *International Journal of Clinical and Experimental Hypnosis, 18,* 235–250.

Spiegel, H., & Bridger, A.A. (1970). *Manual for hypnotic induction profile: Eye-roll levitation method.* New York: Soni Medica.

Spiegel, H., & Spiegel, D. (1978). *Trance and treatment: Clinical uses of hypnosis.* New York: Basic Books.

Tellegen, A., & Atkinson, G. (1974). Openness to absorbing and self-altering experiences ("absorption"), a trait related to hypnotic susceptibility. *Journal of Abnormal Psychology, 83,* 268–277.

Turner, J.A., & Chapman, C.R. (1982). Psychological interventions for chronic pain: A critical review. II. Operant conditioning, hypnosis, and cognitive-behavioral therapy. *Pain, 12,* 23–46.

Unestahl, L.E. (1979). Hypnotic preparation of athletes. In G.D. Burrows, D.R. Collison and L. Dennerstein. *Hypnosis.* New York: Elsevier.

Vingoe, F.J. (1968). The development of a group alert0trance scale. *International Journal of Clinical and Experimental Hypnosis, 16,* 120–132.

Wagstaff, G.F. (1981). *Hypnosis, compliance and belief.* New York: St. Martin's Press.

Weitzenhoffer, A.M. (1957) *General techniques of hypnotism.* New York: Grune and Stratton.

Weitzenhoffer, A.M., & Hilgard, E.R. (1959). *Stanford Hypnotic Susceptibility Scale, Forms A and B.* Palo Alto, CA: Consulting Psychologists Press.

Weitzenhoffer, A.M., & Hilgard, E.R. (1962). *Stanford Hypnotic Susceptibility Scale, Form C.* Palo Alto, CA: Consulting Psychologists Press.

Chapter 2

HYPNOSIS AND THE MANAGEMENT OF CHRONIC PAIN[1]

FREDERICK J. EVANS, PH.D.

The aim of this chapter is to clarify some of the important differences between acute and chronic pain, and to present a rationale for the application of hypnotic techniques for the treatment of acute and chronic pain. The focus is on chronic pain and hypnosis, but it is necessary to understand the way in which acute pain transitions into chronic pain if the core anxiety about the meaning of pain is not successfully managed. Anxiety and worry about the persisting pain turns into (internalized) anger, helplessness and (masked or somatized) depression as the persisting pain becomes unmanageable.

Patients come to see a doctor initially for at least one of three reasons: they have a fever, they are anxious about a symptom of unknown importance, or for up to 80 percent of initial visits, they have pain. Most of the time, the anxiety, fever, or pain is treated successfully. However, in a growing number of patients the pain does not necessarily abate over time. In the 1986 Nuprin report (Sternbach, 1986), it was found that for all United States adults, more than 4 billion work days were lost per year, about 23 days per adult person. In 1986, this translated into a productivity loss of over $55 billion dollars.

---

[1]. PATHFINDERS: Consultants in Human Behavior, 736 Lawrence Road, Lawrenceville, NJ 08648. USA. (Phone and Fax: 609 683 0717 e-mail: AUSSIEDR@AOL>COM). Affiliated with Pain Management Services, Reading Hospital, PA; Pain Management, Medical Center of Princeton, NJ; Pain Care Institute, Philadelphia, Pa and the Back Rehab Institute, Hamilton and Princeton, NJ. I wish to thank George Strobel, MD, Whitney Collins, Ph.D., and Rebecca Tendler, Ph.D. for their critical comments, and Blanche E. Anderson for her editorial help.

SENSORY AND AFFECTIVE COMPONENTS OF PAIN

Even acute pain is not always a simple matter of stimulus intensity in the clinical situation. A college student, Lee S., illustrates this in an autobiographical account. While serving as an infantry squad leader in . . . Vietnam I stepped on a concussion-type . . . land mine and had my left foot twisted to a right angle inward from its normal position at the end of the leg. My boot and sock were totally blown off by the blast of the mine. Upon regaining consciousness and for many days afterwards I felt no pain and in fact experienced euphoria at the thought of leaving Vietnam and returning home. While being carried to the medevac helicopter some forty-five minutes after stepping on the mine, I can recall smiling and even crying with relief during the lift on the guy line to the hovering helicopter. I'm not certain whether I was in a slight state of shock, however I recall carrying out what seems to me to have been a coherent conversation while waiting for the medevac. . . . I was certain I was going to live and I was thankful for that. . . .

After the operation to amputate the injured extremity, I was administered Demerol and shuttled to several hospitals in Vietnam. At one hospital I had a boil removed from my arm which was a slightly painful operation and I now consider this pain of removal primarily due to a perceived delay in what I was beginning to realize was my total removal from the war zone. This minor operation was more of a nuisance and it is interesting to note that as yet I had felt no pain in my stump. . . .

Three weeks later upon regaining consciousness after the second operation but still under sedation, I was terribly upset that I was an amputee and the operation had removed more irreplaceable bone. After speaking to my parents I grew quite anxious to get back to the States and when a doctor removed my bandages for the first time I felt what seemed to be excruciating pain (in spite of continued injections of Demerol). This was perhaps the first realization that I was no longer in Vietnam (and danger) and that I was safe in the care of medical help. I was told that I would be sent home as soon as I was well enough to travel and this knowledge provided the psychological motivation for my experiencing (and acting in) less pain from the dressing changes each day. I was requesting fewer injections and in several days switched to Darvon compound.

From the time I left Japan until after I saw my family, I was in no pain whatsoever. After my family had left the hospital, I had my first experiences of phantom pains or a sensation that the limb was still there. . . .

I received a final operation to join my fibula and tibia together four months after the injury and was actually running in my permanent prosthesis four weeks after surgery. With the exception of slight and occasional experiences of phantom pains during periods of stress, my final four months of hospitalization were relatively free of pain and absolutely without severe pain. At home and at the hospital I was kept by others, or kept myself constantly busy either by others or myself and thus diverted my attention from the disability which I attribute to the lack of noticeable pain. At the hospital it was truly remarkable to witness the correlation between those who were constantly bored, did little, always complained and generally were wallowing in self-pity and the amount of pain they seemed to suffer and perhaps consequently the length of their time to recover."

Similar accounts of the distinction between the sensory and secondary affective components of pain have been documented often before this personal report of a brave man. Wounded soldiers on the Anzio beachhead during World War II typically did not report pain as they waited to be removed from the battlefield, in spite of gunshot and shrapnel wounds that may eventually have needed major surgery, amputation, and long-term convalescence. Beecher (1946, 1959) contrasted the wounded soldier's mild euphoria with similarly injured civilians in a hospital emergency setting, who typically writhed in agony and demanded immediate attention and medication. The soldier knew he was going home, and he no longer had to fear being killed; for the civilian the pain has socioeconomic and emotional implications. Beecher's observations were not new, having been made during the Napoleonic Wars, and in China 2000 years ago (Tan, Tan & Vieth, 1973).

Beecher's (1959) emphasis on how the psychological significance of the injury experience modulates pain severity has led to the delineation of learning factors and early experience in the development of long-term pain behavior (Fordyce, 1976; Sternbach, 1982; Turk, Meichenbaum & Genest, 1983). A young child, after falling, may look around to see if a parent is nearby to provide tender loving care before deciding whether to cry or continue to return to play with his or her friends. Early learning experiences in handling transient pain may develop into an enduring behavioral pattern in which pain and suffering can become instrumental in manipulating the environment (e.g., getting attention from Mommy, receiving the good-tasting cherry-flavored medicine, avoiding school). Learning and adaptation factors are prevalent in the psychological history of chronic pain patients, and may help explain the significance of the secondary gain that is usually evident in the history of chronic pain patients.

DISSOCIATIVE AND PLACEBO COMPONENTS OF HYPNOTIC ANALGESIA

The meticulous psychophysical studies of experimental pain conducted by Hilgard (1969, 1977) and others have shown that there is a lawful relationship between the intensity of the noxious stimulation and the subjective experience of transient, acute pain. The relationship between stimulus intensity and pain reports also holds for the reduction of pain following hypnotic analgesia. In contrast, clinical studies often find little correlation between (chronic) pain reduction and measured hypnotizability (Hilgard, 1977; Large, 1994).

Early studies of hypnotic analgesia measured only pain threshold and carefully made sure that the subject's anxiety was minimized (Shor, 1962). As a result, studies were unable to demonstrate that hypnotic analgesia was effective before the study by McGlashan, Evans, and Orne (1969). The role of anxiety on experimental pain was shown by an elegant demonstration by Orne (1974). He showed that male college students' reports of painful electric shock, which they had rated as strong as they could continue to tolerate, increased dramatically when they were told that some girls from the local high school performed better. Other subjects rated electric shocks to the fingers as much less intense when they were told the study was about skin sensitivity compared to the stronger ratings for same level intensity of shock by students who were told that a new form of current was being used in this study, but the experimenters were fairly certain that the electric shocks would not do any tissue damage.

Meaningful experimental studies relevant to clinical pain are restricted to those pain induction procedures using protracted above threshold measurements such as ischemic pain or cold pressor pain tolerance and endurance levels. In one of the first such studies, McGlashan et al. (1969); (see also Evans, 1984, 1987a, 1990b; Evans & McGlashan, 1987; Hilgard & Hilgard, 1975; Orne, 1974; Wagstaff, 1987) compared hypnotic and placebo analgesia. They used ischemic pain tolerance, which had been shown to be responsive to pain medication and therefore was as reasonable analog for studying experimental pain. They studied 12 extreme high and 12 low hypnotizable subjects whose hypnotic ability was evaluated independently for at least three intensive sessions. Individually, the subjects participated in three sessions: (1) during highly motivated baseline conditions; (2) following the induction of hypnotic analgesia, including a clinically-derived procedure to motivate low hypnotizable subjects to expect some successful hypnotic analgesia; (3) after ingesting a placebo capsule which the experimenter thought was part of a double blind drug study. The "drug" session was legitimized to the subject as a control against which to evaluate the analgesic effects of hypnosis. The logic of this study was to maximize variables influencing the placebo effect, as is done in the clinic, rather than to control or eliminate them, as had been done in traditional experimental studies.

Three aspects of the results were especially important.

1. There was a dramatic increase in pain tolerance for deeply hypnotizable subjects during hypnotically-induced analgesia. This is likely to be a result of the dissociative aspects of the hypnotic condition when it occurs in subjects who are very responsive to hypnosis.

2. The much smaller but significant placebo-induced change in ischemic pain tolerance was equal in magnitude for both high hypnotizable and low hypnotizable subjects.

3. The hypnotic analgesia suggestions significantly improved tolerance of ischemic pain even for low hypnotizable subjects. For these hypnotically unresponsive subjects, the pain relief produced by the placebo component of the hypnotic context and the placebo component of ingesting a pill are about equal, and highly correlated (.76, N =12). This is the "placebo" or expectational component of the hypnotic induction procedure.

The expectation that hypnosis can be helpful in reducing pain produced similar significant reductions in pain as the expectations derived from taking a pain-killing pill, even in those individuals who otherwise have no special hypnotic skills. Significant pain relief was achieved under both the placebo analgesia and placebo hypnosis conditions,

PAIN TOLERANCE INCREASE WITH HYPNOSIS AND PLACEBO

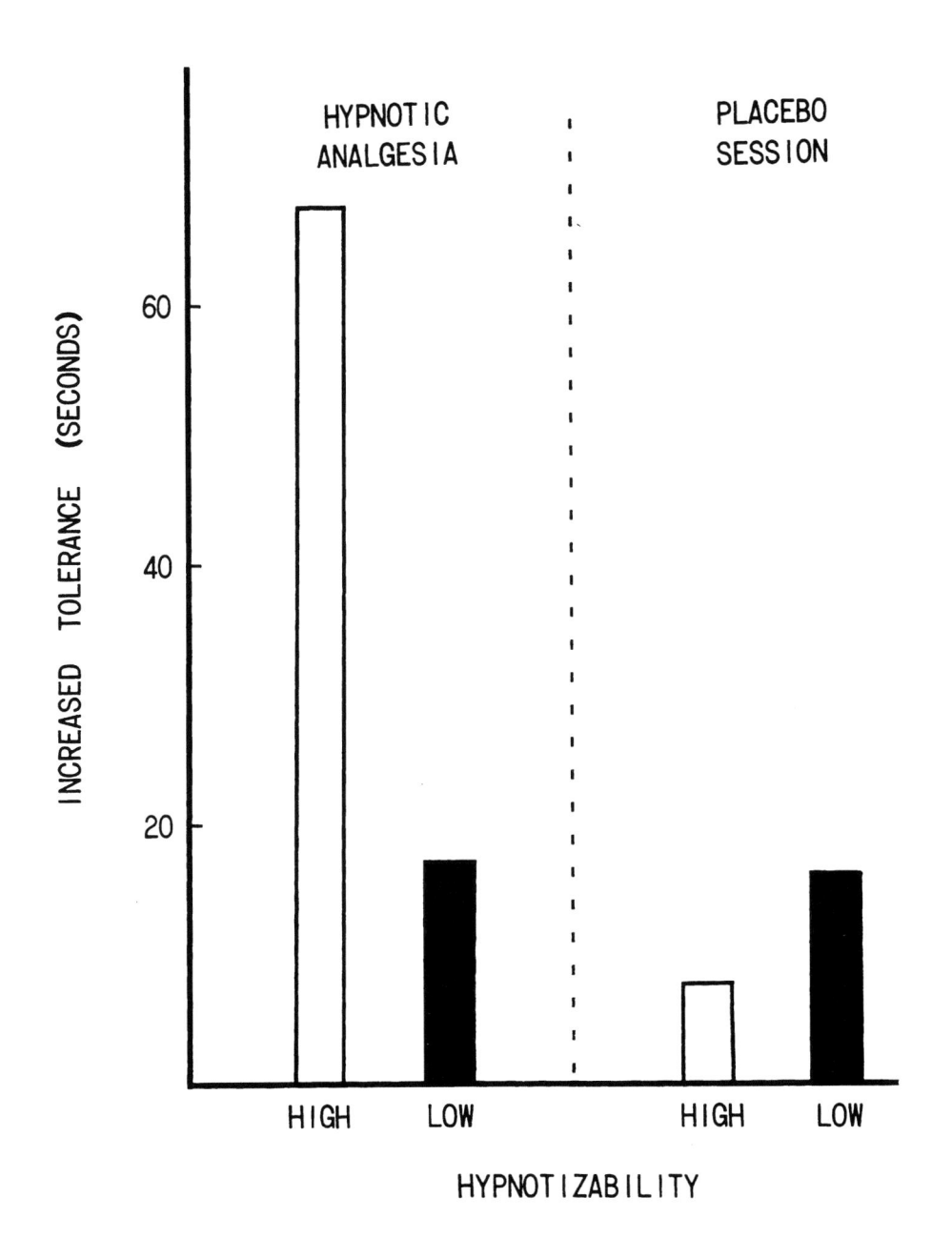

Figure 2-1. Comparison of high and low hypnotizable subjects (n=12, 12) on the increased tolerance of ischemic pain under conditions of hypnotic analgesia and ingestion of a placebo pill

even though this relief was not nearly as great as that obtained with hypnotic analgesia in highly hypnotizable subjects.

This study shows that the mechanisms by which a placebo pill and hypnosis produced analgesia were different in subjects with high hypnotic capacity. Several studies using different methodologies have produced similar results. For example, Knox, Gekoski, Shum, and McLaughlin (1981) compared acupuncture with hypnosis. The pain reduction with acupuncture was equal in high and low hypnotizable subjects, but the pain response of highly hypnotizable subjects was significantly greater with hypnosis than with acupuncture.[2] Miller and Bowers (1986) found a similar result in a study in which Meichenbaum's (1977) stress inoculation procedure was compared to hypnotic analgesia.

In summary, then, these studies and others show that hypnosis can facilitate a number of cognitive strategies that can be helpful in alleviating acute experimental pain. Specific interventions such as acupuncture, attention/distraction, pain medication, placebo, relaxation, and stress inoculation have significant effects on pain, but these effects seem to be independent of individual differences in hypnotic capacity (Evans, 1989). The label "hypnosis" produces a powerful, almost magical, connotation that *change* is expected. The expectation of therapeutic success may be strong in the therapist as well as in the patient, and is uncorrelated with the patient's hypnotizability. The confident communications to the patient that help is on its way are powerful therapeutic interventions that cannot be overlooked in treating pain. The magical connotations of "hypnosis" and the ritual of the hypnotic induction process produce powerful nonspecific therapeutic effects that may lead to substantial pain control in many patients, even those with limited hypnotic capacity. In this sense, as many clinicians claim, hypnosis may work for everybody, except the treatment-resistant

---

2. The magnitude of this nonspecific response can be considerable. For patients who reduce clinical pain following a placebo injection, about 95% will also respond to a standard dose of morphine. However, in those patients who do not reduce pain following a placebo trial, only about 50% respond to morphine (Lasagna, Mosteller, Von Felsinger & Beecher, 1954). Evans (1984, 1985) showed that the relative effectiveness of placebo compared to a standard dose of morphine is about 56% in double-blind studies. The placebo is also from 50% to 60% as effective as aspirin, codeine, and Darvon, as well as for nonpain treatments, including the pharmacological and behavioral treatment of insomnia and the double-blind use of lithium in psychiatric patients. This implies that the nonspecific factors arising from the treatment milieu are important clinical variables, presumably operating because the therapist communicates his enthusiasm and expectations of success to the suffering patient.

patient, even though for some, the clinical effects are produced by the context of hypnosis rather than the hypnotic condition itself.

On the other hand, these studies show that for some highly hypnotizable individuals, hypnosis provided control and mastery of pain that is different from procedures such as placebo (Evans, 1984, 1985, in press, a), acupuncture (Knox, Gekoski, Shum, McGlaughlin, 1981), biofeedback (Melzack & Perry, 1975), stress inoculation (Miller & Bowers, 1986), and naloxone-induced biochemical changes (Goldstein & Grevert, 1978; Spiegel & Albert, 1983). Just as in the studies of the interaction between placebo response and morphine response (Beecher, 1959; Evans, 1985), these interpersonal and individual trait aspects of hypnosis cannot easily be separated. Only the trait components depend on measured hypnotic skill.

The fact that there are at least two interacting mechanisms involved helps to explain why clinicians often see compelling pain relief in patients treated by hypnosis who otherwise seem unhypnotizable by adequate measurement. The capacity to experience hypnosis may be a powerful bonus, but the nonspecific components of the hypnotic situation may also provide powerful therapeutic leverage. If hypnosis is useful with chronic pain cases where depression and secondary gain are the key therapeutic issues, it is likely to involve these nonspecific aspects of the hypnotic context as well as hypnotic capacity.[3]

HYPNOSIS AND CHRONIC PAIN: REVIEW OF STUDIES

Clinical reports document that hypnosis has been used to reduce chronic pain (Sacerdote, 1970), to reduce the pain and severity of debridement procedures in burn patients (Ewin, 1979), and to assist in the management of pain in the terminally ill cancer patient (Domangue & Margolis, 1983). There are relatively few well-controlled empirical studies of the clinical efficacy of hypnosis in the management of acute or chronic pain (Turner & Chapman, 1982). The evidence suggests that about 50 percent of terminal cancer patients (Hilgard & Hilgard, 1975) and 95 percent of dental patients (J.

---

3. Acupuncture and hypnosis involve different mechanisms. Studies have shown that the opiate antagonist Naloxone reverses the pain alleviation of acupuncture and other pain reducing strategies but does not affect the pain reduction produced by hypnosis (Goldstein & Hilgard, 1975; Spiegel & Albert, 1983; Wagstaff, 1987; Evans & McGlashan, 1987).

Barber, 1977) can be helped with some pain control by the adjunctive use of hypnotic techniques. Recently, a powerful policy statement was issued by the National Institutes of Health Technology Conference (1995) on "The Integration of Behavioral and Relaxation Approaches into the Treatment of Chronic Pain and Insomnia," finding that "hypnosis is effective in alleviating chronic pain associated with various cancers... (and) irritable bowel syndrome, inflammatory conditions of the mouth, temporomandibular disorders, and tension headaches." Large (1994) and Holroyd (1996) have reviewed most of the studies which led to this conclusion.

Studying mixed groups of chronic pain patients, Melzack and Perry (1975) found that a combination of hypnosis and biofeedback was more effective in alleviating pain than either technique alone (N=24). Elton, Burrows, and Stanley (1980) found that hypnosis was more effective than behavioral therapy and pill placebo with 30 chronic pain patients. James, Large, and Beale (1989) effectively individualized self-hypnotic strategies in five chronic pain patients using a multiple baseline study.

Crasilneck (1979) found 69 percent of 29 consecutive low back pain referrals reported 80 percent subjective pain relief during outpatient treatment with individualized hypnosis lasting up to 9 months. McCauley, Thelen, Frank, Willard, and Callen (1983) found positive results for both hypnosis and relaxation with back pain patients.

Two studies have shown the effectiveness of hypnosis with painful irritable bowel syndrome. Whorwell, Prior, and Faragher (1984) found hypnosis reduced subjective pain and abdominal distension in 30 patients compared to supportive psychotherapy. This group (Prior, Colgan & Whorwell, 1990) later found that hypnosis reduced rectal sensitivity in 15 diarrhea prone patients.

Compared to physical therapy, hypnosis was more effective in improving pain and sleep, but not tender points, in 40 patients with fibromyalgia (Haanen, Hoenderdos, vanRomunde, Hop, Mallee, Terwiel & Hekster, 1991). Medication reduction was observed in 80 percent of the patients treated with hypnosis. Several anecdotal reports (Margolis, personal communication; Finer, personal communication; Gainer, 1992; Evans & Strobel, in progress) suggest that hypnosis might be effective in the early phases of reflex sympathetic dystrophy, but formal studies have not yet been completed.

In one of the few studies that measured hypnotic ability, Stam,

McGrath, and Brooke (1984) found that the more highly hypnotizable of 61 patients with temporomandibular joint pain gained relief with both hypnosis and relaxation compared to a control group. There was little pain reduction with any of the treatments for low hypnotizable patients.

Syrjala, Cummings, and Donaldson (1992) found that hypnosis was more effective than cognitive behavioral therapy in reducing pain, but not nausea, emesis, nor opioid use in 67 bone marrow transplant patients. This result is a little surprising in view of the widely held anecdotal reports that hypnosis is an excellent tool for treating nausea and vomiting in several clinical populations, including hyperemesis in early pregnancy, bulimia, and treatment-induced emesis in cancer patients (Evans, 1991).

Several studies have shown the value of hypnosis treating chronic headache. Olness, MacDonald, and Uden (1987) found hypnosis was superior to propranolol or placebo in treating 28 children with migraine headaches. Cedercreutz (1976) treated 100 patients with severe migraine headaches using hypnosis. Of the 55 percent of patients whose migraines decreased over three months, most were highly hypnotizable. It is not clear what measure of hypnotic ability was used, nor were there any control groups. Basker, Anderson, and Dalton (1976) compared 47 patients with migraine headaches randomly assigned to hypnosis or drug (prochlorperazine). Complete remission over three months occurred in significantly more of the hypnotized patients (43%) compared to the drug group (12%). At least three studies (N=55, 56, 79) from Holland (vanDyck, Zitman, Linssen & Spinhoven, 1991; Spinhoven, Linssen, vanDyck & Zitman, 1991; Zitman, vanDyck, Spinhoven & Linssen, vanDyck & Zitman, 1992) have found that hypnosis or self-hypnosis, especially among the more hypnotizable, reduces tension headache pain, at least as well as autogenic training, and better than in control groups.

This is not a comprehensive nor critical review of existing studies. No attempt has been made to review studies using hypnosis in the treatment of cancer pain, such as the recent work of Spiegel (1993). It is intended to show that hypnosis may be one valuable technique to help reduce chronic pain of various origins. These studies use a wide variety of hypnotic techniques, and they do not indicate which hypnotic strategies might be more helpful for specific painful conditions. Most of the studies lack appropriate control groups and have inadequate follow up data (at least two years of follow-up is necessary). Several of the studies find no difference in efficacy between hypnosis and other active psychosocial treatment modalities, but some show that hypnosis can be as effective as direct medical interventions (e.g., pain medication). Unfortunately, hypnotic ability is rarely related to outcome, neither in the hypnosis nor the comparison groups. Therefore it is not known if the pain reduction is due to the specific effects of high hypnotic ability or to nonspecific effects associated with the use of hypnotic interventions. Nor do these studies come to terms with the difficult issue of how best to measure pain reduction. Most have been forced to rely on subjective pain ratings of unknown reliability. The clinical criterion of successful treatment outcome for chronic pain patients if far more complex than mere pain reduction. Multiple outcome measures need to consider decreased depression, medication and opioid use; improved sleep; weight gain; social and family relations; quality of life; increase in range of motion and activity level; and return to work (Eimer & Freeman, 1998; Evans, 1989; Fordyce, 1976; Sternbach, 1968; Turk, Meichenbaum & Genest, 1982).

USE OF HYPNOSIS IN DIFFERENT TYPES OF PAIN

Table 2-1 provides a useful roadmap to help guide the adjunctive use of various hypnosis techniques in acute pain, headache, and chronic pain with and without a clear organic or anatomical basis. It summarizes the way in which hypnosis is used in the type of pain, the time course of treatment, and the goals of hypnotic interventions, and comments on anticipated additional benefits to the patient from the use of hypnosis (the so-called "ripple" effect). These summary statements will be expanded throughout the chapter.

Cancer and Terminal Pain Patients

Hypnosis is often dramatic in helping the cancer patient control pain, although it usually does not eliminate it completely. Hypnosis can help in reducing medication, controlling nausea and vomiting and the side effects of chemotherapy (Domangue & Margolis, 1983), and minimizing the threat of needles, bone marrow tests, and other invasive procedures, especially in children (Olness, 1998). Cancer patients with excessive nausea and vomiting are usually very responsive to

TABLE 2-1

THE ADJUNCTIVE USE OF HYPNOSIS IN THE TREATMENT OF DIFFERENT TYPES OF PAIN.

Summary of pain type, treatment goals and secondary benefits of the use of hypnotic techniques.

Type of pain	Typical use of hypnosis	Time course	Treatment goals	Secondary effects
Acute Pain	Relaxation/anxiety reduction	Very short-term, often crisis intervention	Reduce anxiety, provide support	Increase accessibility to appropriate treatment
Cancer Pain	Self-hypnosis, often with relaxation and imagery	Very short-term, with "booster" sessions	Teach patient to suffer less with dignity	Reduction in nausea and other side effects of treatment
Chronic Pain: clear organic pathology	Self-hypnosis, usually directed at symptom, imagery and focused attention	Multiple sessions as needed	Teach self-control and mastery experiences	Reduction in suffering and improved ego strength due to self-control
Chronic Pain: no clear organic basis	Self-hypnosis and dissociative skills	Short-term aggressive. Long-term psychological and/or pharmacological therapy	Short-term: control body function, e.g., glove analgesia. Learn self-control. Long-term: secondary gain, depression	Management of underlying depression
Headache	Varies based on type: relaxation, self-control, tension reduction, imagery	Variable, often with "booster" sessions	Symptom reduction, strategies for quality of life, as needed	Stress and tension reduction and self-control skills

Assumes thorough medical, psychological and diagnostic evaluation, and hypnosis used within the limits of professional training and competence.

hypnosis. Imagery techniques work very well. These patients can usually learn rapid self-hypnotic techniques that are then available to them whenever needed (see Table 2-1).

There are two important warnings for the therapist using hypnosis in this context. First, the improvement in the patient's functioning is easily misinterpreted as the remission of the cancer, and some family therapy is needed to clarify for parties that hypnosis is being used to help the patient to suffer less, and with dignity, rather than to produce a cure. Second, the self-hypnosis procedures usually work—for a while. After days, or even weeks, self-hypnosis often loses effectiveness. This may coincide with stressors such as a new medical report, or a change in treatment, or a family dispute. Fortunately, relatively rapid "booster" sessions with the therapist will usually reestablish the effectiveness of self-hypnosis. If a brief hypnotic technique, such as the Eye Roll technique (Evans, in press (b); see Chapter 1), is well practiced, sometimes these boosters can be conducted quickly by telephone contact during the therapist's telephone hour.

Acute Pain and Hypnosis

The management of acute pain primarily involves the management of anxiety. The growing anxiety about the short- and long-term consequences of the injury that accompanies the increasing intensity of the acute noxious stimulation is usually relieved by adequate treatment (e.g., pain medication, hypnosis, or other interventions to reduce anxiety). Many experimental studies have shown (Turner & Chapman, 1982) a clear relationship between increases in anxiety and increases in pain intensity. Although there are no studies documenting it, it is clinically accepted that the reverse will hold: reduction in anxiety will automatically be followed by reduction in reported pain. Hypnosis is a simple and effective method of reducing anxiety either by direct suggestions or by any technique that helps the patient relax. Level of hypnotic responsivity is usually irrelevant, and the response is likely due to the nonspecific components of the hypnotic procedure (expectation of relief promised). In an emergency injury with resulting pain, the mere whispered soft, slow intonation of a hypnotic relaxation procedure is a dramatic contrast to the decibel level usually associated with an anxious visit to the emergency room. If the sufferer has sufficient hypnotic talent, secondary effects are possible. These include the control of bleeding, reduced medication, and relaxation necessary for emergency medical intervention including minor surgery and suturing.

Similar uses of hypnosis are often extremely effective in treating burns and making debridement procedures more tolerable (Patterson, Adcock & Bombardier, 1997), and with minor surgery itself! The management of headaches has components of all the pain types in Table 2-1. Pain due to cancer, burn, and surgery will be explored more fully in other chapters of this book.

It should be noted that patients with high levels of anxiety occasionally react counterexpectationally to relaxation methods. They may become even more anxious. These patients may respond well to imagery techniques and active hypnotic procedures. They may relax if they are allowed to leave their eyes open, or if they are positively assured that they will not lose self-control during hypnosis.

FROM ACUTE PAIN TO CHRONIC PAIN: ANXIETY TO DEPRESSION

The management of acute pain primarily involves the management of anxiety. When the acute pain is not relieved satisfactorily, a different set of dynamics arises as another more chronic pattern becomes established. Although pain intensity may have increased initially, it tends to abate gradually, but the fear of continued suffering remains. The anticipatory fear of continuing pain gives way to a frightening awareness that a painful injury or lesion may have a more permanent effect. The transition is expressed by the acute feeling that "My God, it *hurts!*" to the transitional "*Oh!* My God it still hurts, what now?" to the long-term "*Oh,* My God!" Despair and despondency gradually develop as the suffering remains unrelieved, and activities become restricted. Gradually, a time-protracted pattern is established involving helplessness and depression that reinforces pain behavior (Fordyce, 1976; Sternbach, 1968). The pain may be experienced at a site remote from the original injury site (such as in fibromyalgia or in reflex sympathetic dystrophy).

Feelings of helplessness lead to depression, guilt, and internalized anger concerning perceived loss of bodily parts or functions, and diminished self-control. Seeking, demanding, and receiving help from significant others, including parents, spouses, children, friends, and doctors, and the mildly pleasant and/or euphoric effects of medication, or the sedation by which sleep avoids the pain, all produce a seductive reinforcement contingency for which the pain is a sufficient, and eventually a necessary experience. This is the source of the secondary gain that often temporarily limits the use of hypnotic interventions.

Pain is sometimes positively reinforced by its pleasant consequences, and sometimes negative consequences are avoided by continued pain. Good things happen only when the patient has pain. "My low back pain allows me to watch the Sunday football game instead of mowing the lawn." "The pain medicine makes me forget all about the suffering."

Pain prevents bad things from happening. "When I have my migraines, I can avoid my spouse's advances, and my impossible kids go outside and play." "My poor spouse will not leave me while I am still suffering." To paraphrase Henry Higgins, "the gain in pain is mostly in the brain." The use of hypnosis in these patients may be helpful, but different strategies are necessary. Early hypnotic intervention based on anxiety reduction, relaxation, or symptom removal will only frustrate the patient and the therapist and will usually be unsuccessful. For the occasional chronic pain patient for whom hypnosis does reduce pain directly before the patient has resolved the emotional effects of the pain, increased depression and occasionally suicidal ideation may occur. The use of hypnosis in chronic pain patients may be helpful, but different strategies are needed, usually later in the therapy. It is appropriate to consider that any chronic pain patient is depressed until proven otherwise, especially when there is no apparent somatic or organic basis to the pain. When using hypnosis for pain control, it is necessary to address simultaneously the depression and secondary gain as psychotherapeutic issues. Early in treatment, hypnosis will usually be restricted to the introduction of mind-body, self-control techniques not directly related to the pain (see Chapter 1 for some useful techniques).

CLINICAL ASSESSMENT OF CHRONIC PAIN

The typical chronic pain patient will have unsuccessfully experienced an average of five previous treatment modalities before coming to a therapist who uses hypnosis. These will often have included neurologists and neurosurgeons ("when in doubt, cut it out"), manipulative procedures by orthopedic and chiropractic specialists ("when in doubt, pound it out"), psychological interventions ("when in doubt, talk it out"), and extensive pharmacological interventions ("when in doubt, medicate"). Many chronic pain patients will have been involved in psychological and psychiatric treatment (or should be), and have sought input from other well-meaning sources, including spouses, lovers, friends, and the local hairdresser. Partly because of the patient's pain-emergent depression and internalized anger, the clinician is usually discouraged and the initial confrontation is often an adversarial one (Sternbach, 1968). The patient's demand is to "help poor me, doc" (when the implicit meaning is "I know you can't"), "fix me up" ("you're probably another quack"), and "write me another prescription" ("I need to maintain my addiction"). These negative beliefs are not conducive to a meaningful therapeutic relationship. Chronic pain patients feel that dealing with doctors, attorneys, and insurance companies is like having a full-time job.

For many of these patients, the demand "hypnotize me and get rid of my pain" is often an invitation to failure. When the burden of cure is abrogated to an assumed magical technique like hypnosis, which may be seen as a last resort for a cure, any initial attempt to use hypnosis will at best be unsuccessful and at worst precipitate an early termination of the therapeutic encounter.

The initial therapeutic contract is very important when hypnosis is to be used with the chronic pain patient. The therapist will often use a firm, direct, confrontational style in order to evaluate the depression, somatization, and secondary gain issues quickly, because these issues will determine the focus of the treatment plan. Four direct questions summarized in Table 2-2 are often helpful to achieve this.

1. *What difference would it make to your life if suddenly you had no pain?* The response to this question is often hedged with anger and impatience. It will reveal hints about the psychic utility of the pain as a reinforcement system. For example, consider the implications of the response: "Oh, I would have to go back to my goddamned traveling salesman job and be away from my family most of the time."

2. *Do you want to get better?* Patients with chronic pain masking depression will rarely give an unequivocal "yes" to this question. An angry "What do you mean? Of course, I want to get better!" is a typ-

TABLE 2-2

KEY QUESTIONS FOR EVALUATING PAIN PATIENTS

Pain Severity Rating

On a one to ten scale, where "one" is no pain at all and "ten" is the worst pain you could imagine anyone ever having, how would you rate your pain now?

This is a general scale, like the often-used visual analog scales used by others that can be modified in various ways, e.g., *"What is the worst (best) your pain gets?" "What would you rate the pain now?"* (before, after treatment, etc.). Can be used at any time during treatment.

Evaluating Secondary Gain and Depression

1. *What difference would it make to your life if suddenly you had no pain?*
2. *Do you want to get better?*

   Repeat the question up to three time until an unequivocal "yes" is obtained. Make special note of any answer other than a simple "yes" or "of course I do."

Establishing the Therapeutic Contract

Ascertain current pain rating. Assume, for example, patient says "8."

3. *If we were successful in reducing your pain from an _____ to about _____ (4, half the current level), would you be satisfied?*

4. *Will you work hard with me to get better?*

Evaluating Self-Esteem

What do you like about yourself?

(Record time in seconds until patient begins answering)

What don't you like about yourself?

Other Clinically Useful Questions

What color is your pain?
What is your favorite color?
What shape is your pain?
If you were an animal, what would you be?

ical response. This question should be repeated three times, giving the patient an opportunity to give a simple "yes" response. Failure to obtain a sincere "yes" usually indicates a poor prognosis. Depressed patients will quickly become more angry and frustrated with repetition of this question. Patients who give a simple unqualified "yes" to this question are unlikely to have significant emotional and secondary gain issues, and in these cases, direct interventions to reduce pain with hypnosis can proceed and will usually be successful (see Table 2-2, also Evans, 1989, 1999, in press).

3. *Would you be satisfied if your pain could be reduced by about half?* This is both a contractual and informational question exploring whether the patient has realistic expectations about pain relief. Patients who can accept partial relief as a goal have more realistic expectations about outcome. This question is easy to ask using the 1 to 10 pain rating scale summarized in Table 2-2.

4. *Are you willing to work hard to get better?* This question is useful to explain to the patient that the therapist may not have a magical cure, and that hypnosis will probably help, but it does not guarantee dramatic results. The emphasis is on the ability of the patient to work at getting better rather than expecting the therapist to produce some effortless "quick fix." The importance of practicing short and long self-hypnosis exercises can be pointed out in this context (see Chapter 1 for some sample transcripts).

If the answers to these four direct questions are unsatisfactory, it may be necessary to tell patients who cannot accept the basic therapeutic contract that this approach may not be right for them, and that perhaps they should be treated with other modalities. The clinician then has to make a difficult decision: continue therapy with a patient with a poor prognostic outcome or refer the patient elsewhere, who may then seek help from another source that may be harmful, such as further surgery, more dangerous medications, or resorting to possibly harmful unproven techniques.[4] These questions also provide a useful transition to discuss misconceptions about hypnosis and to emphasize that the responsibility for improvement rests with the patient rather

---

4. For the minority of chronic patient patients who give direct and simple answers to these questions, secondary gain and depression are not likely to be involved in the pain dynamics. Any hypnotic intervention can be safe and useful with these patients immediately in therapy for pain management.

than with the therapist. The therapist's role as a special and powerful teacher, mentor, or facilitator is emphasized.

The way in which the patient is asked to describe his or her pain may be very useful later to help select appropriate imagery and cognitive strategies when it is time to use hypnotic interventions. Many patients find it difficult to describe their pain verbally but can complete written instruments such as the McGill Pain Questionnaire (Melzack, 1975) or the Multiphasic Pain Inventory (Rudy, 1989), or other assessment techniques summarized in Turk and Melzack (1992) or Eimer and Freeman (1998). Techniques such as drawing or painting the pain, describing the color and shape of the pain, and exploring conditions under which it is more or less intense (heat, cold, sitting) may be relevant to help develop treatment strategies. Asking the patient to name the pain, and then write a letter to the pain (using an uncensored, mindlessness set, stream-of-consciousness mental set, or dissociative style, possibly during hypnosis) will provide clues as to how to manage internalized anger. Patients need help with how to deal with anger about their pain using techniques, sometimes facilitated with self-hypnosis, such as exercise, humor, projective methods such as writing, drawing, or working on crafts and hobbies, and especially safe fantasy and imagery.

SOME HYPNOTIC TECHNIQUES FOR CHRONIC PAIN

Several techniques (Evans, 1987a, 1989) are useful to help the patient "discover" that he or she is capable of controlling bodily sensations, especially pain. Suggested glove analgesia can be induced in all except a few resistant patients. If this is done with care, the patient gradually begins to believe that he or she can control physiological or somatic experiences in a part of his or her body. With repeated experience, glove analgesia can be transferred to the pain-afflicted area, but this should be done cautiously with due regard for the patient's secondary gain issues.

Imagery, relaxation, and self-hypnotic methods are usually introduced. Use of the Chevreul pendulum will help circumvent resistance. A crystal, washer, or key is suspended about 15 inches on a thread, and held by the patient between the thumb and middle finger, with the elbow resting comfortably on the knee. Suggestions are given to imagine the pendulum swinging back and forth, back and forth, like a pendulum. After about 90 seconds, the suggestion is given to let it slow down, and to swing to and fro, in the opposite direction. After another 90 seconds, it is suggested that it will swing clockwise or counter clockwise or diagonally: the patient should decide which. If the patient is still uncertain who is controlling the pendulum, the patient or therapist, I will encourage the patient to take it home and practice. Almost all patients respond unless deliberately resisting. This is a most engaging and convincing way to introduce the patient to the use of ideomotor suggestion and is an elegant way to introduce the mind-body connection, which usually plays such an important role in later hypnotic interventions with pain patients. Several similar techniques borrowed from sports medicine applications (Unesthal, 1980) are helpful. For example, visual mental rehearsal of getting out of bed for 30–60 seconds before arising will stimulate action potentials that will help the patient quickly overcome the stiffness often experienced when inactive for a period of time. (A sample script for this approach is presented in Chapter 1.)

In the subsequent hypnosis sessions, a delicate balance is required between the initial, authoritarian, direct approach by the therapist to teach the patient mind-body control and the later nondirective cognitive discovery of success. Mastery of physical control in unrelated bodily areas will gradually be discovered insightfully by the patient as relevant to subsequent pain control but only after other issues are resolved in treatment. These issues are usually related to secondary gain, possible posttraumatic stress, medication management and compliance, anger, family and social relationships, medico-legal problems, and activities of everyday living. Teaching self-hypnosis is important. Simple techniques to help relax and manage stress can be taught in early sessions, and any success with some minimal pain reduction is noted. At the same time, this progress must be sufficiently slow so that the patient can be drawn into the therapeutic alliance to handle the psychological issues that are more relevant than the pain experience (e.g., "What if I don't win the compensation case?" "How do I handle my spouse's sexual advances and the children's behavior?").

It is the melody rather than the lyrics that are important in hypnotic techniques. The hypnotic procedures need to be a comfortable mix of the patient's abilities and the therapist's style. Many examples of hypnotic pain reduction suggestions have been outlined by Hammond

(1990, pp. 45-49). Another list of useful techniques covering suggestive, cognitive (imagery and relaxation), and dissociative approaches for pain control is presented in Table 2-3. Most of these techniques listed are easily available in several texts on hypnosis (Crasilneck & Hall, 1979; Hammond, 1990; Hunter, 1994).

The emphasis of these hypnotic interventions is on the mind-body interaction, learning of mastery experiences, and hypnotic facilitation of self-control. However, it is especially important that the patient has permission not to use these mastery techniques in all situations. For example, in a litigation case, a contract can be established (usually while under hypnosis) that the pain can be controlled using hypnosis, but the patient should feel comfortable about deciding when to use these mastery techniques. The tactic of allowing the patient a choice as to when to control pain is an important way to handle the problems associated with the exposure to psychological threat, and the removal of the pain as a defensive reaction. The focus of this kind of hypnotic intervention is to teach the patient that he or she is capable of controlling pain and the related psychological and emotional issues but not to become involved in the ethical and moral issues as to when the patient should use these techniques. Such contracts allow the patient to manipulate pain when it is psychologically appropriate and to progress at his or her own pace. They also provide time to develop a therapeutic alliance and to treat depression if present either with antidepressant medication or appropriate therapeutic techniques.[5]

SUMMARY

The specific applications of hypnosis in pain management will be different depending on the nature and history of the patient's pain. Acute pain is best managed by anxiety-reducing strategies often facilitated by hypnosis. Chronic pain has gradually become a weapon in the control of contingencies in the sufferer's interaction with the internal and external world. It requires strategies that deal with handling one's psychological environment effectively. In such cases, the pain may have no clear organic basis, even though from the patient's view-

---

5. Drug withdrawal if appropriate will be handled slowly in the early sessions. It can be held for later sessions after some of the secondary gain and depression issues are resolved.

TABLE 2-3
SOME HYPNOTIC TECHNIQUES FOR PAIN CONTROL

Early Direct Interventions

    Chevreul Pendulum
    Ego strengthening
    Guided imagery and metaphor
    Mind/body control techniques
    Positive self-suggestion
    Relaxation (breathing, diaphragmatic breathing, progressive relaxation)
    Self-hypnosis
    Spaghetti toes
    Time projection (safe places in the near future)
    What color is your pain?

Ideomotor Techniques

    Ideomotor rehearsal (the mind/body influence)
    Mental rehearsal techniques (sports psychology approaches to pain)
    Triggers and posthypnotic suggestions
    Unconscious signaling (psychodynamic exploration)

Body Dissociation and Self-Control

    Analgesia, glove anesthesia
    Hallucinated pain, and its removal
    Gradual diminution of pain
    Pain displacement
    Reinterpretation of pain signals
    Symptom substitution
    Temperature changes
    Transfer of glove analgesia

Advanced Dissociative Techniques

    Dual video imagery
    Fantasy (for anger management)
    Letters to and from "Mr. Pain"
    Inner adviser, inner creature approaches
    Mystical experiences
    Regression, ideomotor signaling for unconscious exploration of causation

point, "it hurts." Several powerful hypnotic strategies—relaxation, imagery, ideomotor action, dissociation, and self-hypnosis—are available to teach self-control and cognitive mastery.

Further research and controlled clinical trials are necessary to evaluate which of these approaches are most helpful to individual patients with different kinds of persistent pain. However, as each patient suffers in his or her own private way, clinical sensitivity must always take priority over general guidelines for these difficult and misunderstood patients.

REFERENCES

Basker, M.A., Anderson, J.A.D., & Dalton J. (1976). Migraine and hypnotherapy. In F.H. Frankel & H.S. Zamansky (Eds.), *Hypnosis at its bicentennial*. New York: Plenum Press.

Beecher, H.K. (1946). Pain in men wounded in battle. *Annals of Surgery, 123*, 98–105.

Beecher, H.K. (1959). *Measurement of subjective responses: Quantitative effects of drugs*. New York: Oxford University Press.

Bowers, K.S. (1976). *Hypnosis for the seriously curious*. New York: W.W. Norton & Co.

Cedercreutz, C. (1976). Hypnotic treatment of 100 cases of migraine. In F.H. Frankel & H.S. Zamansky (Eds.), *Hypnosis at its bicentennial*. New York: Plenum Press.

Crasilneck, H.B. (1979). Hypnosis in the control of chronic low back pain. *American Journal of Clinical Hypnosis, 22*, 71–81.

Domangue, B.B., & Margolis, C.G. (1983). Hypnosis and a multidisciplinary cancer pain management team: Role and effects. *International Journal of Clinical and Experimental Hypnosis, 31*, 206–212.

Eimer, B.E., & Freeman, A. (1998). *Pain management therapy: A practical guide*. New York: Wiley.

Elton, D., Burrows, G.D., & Stanley, G.V. (1980). Chronic pain and hypnosis. In G.D. Burrows & L. Dennerstein (Eds.), *Handbook of hypnosis and psychosomatic medicine*. Amsterdam: Elsevier/North Holland Biomedical Press.

Esdaile, J. (1957). *Hypnosis in medicine and surgery*. New York: Julian Press. (Originally titled *Mesermism in India*, 1850).

Evans, F.J. (1984). Hypnosis, chronic pain. *Advances: Journal of the Institute for the Advancement of Health, 5*, 11–20.

Evans, F.J. (1985). Expectancy, therapeutic instructions, and the placebo response. In L. White, B. Tursky, & G. Schwartz (Eds.), *Placebo: Clinical phenomena and new insights*. New York: The Guilford Press.

Evans, F.J. (1987a). Hypnosis and chronic pain. In G.D. Burrows, D. Elton, & R. Stanley (Eds.), *Handbook of chronic pain management*. Amsterdam: Elsevier, Amsterdam.

Evans, F.J. (1987b). The hypnotizable patient. Invited Address presented at the IVth

European Congress of Hypnosis and Psychosomatic Medicine, Oxford, England.

Evans, F.J. (1989). Hypnosis. In C.D. Tollison & M.L. Kriegel, (Eds.) *Interdisciplinary rehabilitation of low back pain.* Baltimore: Williams & Wilkins.

Evans, F.J. (1990a). Chronic pain and depression. *Houston Medicine, 6,* 99-103.

Evans, F.J. (1990b). Hypnosis and pain control. *Australian Journal of Clinical and Experimental Hypnosis, 18,* 21-33.

Evans, F.J. (1991). Hypnotizability: Individual differences in dissociation and the flexible control of psychological processes. In S.J. Lynn & J.W. Rhue (Eds.), *Theories of hypnosis.* New York: Gulford.

Evans, F.J. (1999). Hypnosis and the control of pain. *Journal of the International Society of Life Information Science, 17.*

Evans, F.J. (in press). Hypnosis in chronic pain management. In G.D. Burrows, R.G. Stanley, & P.B. Bloom (Eds.). A*dvances in Clinical Hypnosis.* New York, Wiley.

Evans, F.J., & McGlashan, T.H. (1987). Specific and nonspecific factors in hypnotic analgesia: A reply to Wagstaff. *British Journal of Experimental and Clinical Hypnosis, 4,* 141-147.

Ewin, D.M. (1976). Clinical use of Hypnosis for attenuation of burn depth. In F.H. Frankel & H.S. Zamansky (Eds.), *Hypnosis at its bicentennial.* New York: Plenum Press.

Fordyce, W.E. (1976). *Behavioral methods for chronic pain and illness.* St. Louis, MO: C.V. Mosby.

Gainer, M.J. (1992). Hypnotherapy for reflex sympathetic dystrophy. *American Journal of Clinical Hypnosis, 34,* 227-232.

Goldstein, E., & Hilgard, E.R. (1975). Failure of opiate antagonist naloxone to modify hypnotic analgesia. *Proceedings of the National Academy of Science,* U.S.A. 72, 2041-2043.

Haanen, H.C.M., Hoenderdos, H.T.W., vanRomunde, L.K.J., Hop, W.C.J., Mallee, C., Terwiel, J.P., and Hekster, G.B. (1991). Controlled trial of hypnotherapy in the treatment of refractory fibromyalgia. *Journal of Rheumatology, 18,* 72-75.

Hammond, D.C. (Ed.). (1990). *Handbook of hypnotic suggestions and metaphors.* New York: Norton.

Hilgard, E.R. (1965). *Hypnotic susceptibility.* New York: Harcourt, Brace & World.

Hilgard, E.R. (1969). Pain as a puzzle for psychology and physiology. *American Psychologist, 24,* 103-113.

Hilgard, E.R. (1977). *Divided consciousness: Multiple controls in human thought and action.* New York: John Wiley & Sons.

Hilgard, E.R., & Hilgard, J.R. (1975). *Hypnosis in the relief of pain.* Los Altos, CA: William Kaufman, Inc.

Holroyd, J. (1976). Hypnosis treatment of clinical pain. Understanding why hypnosis is useful. *International Journal of Clinical and Experimental Hypnosis, 44,* 33-51.

Hunter, M.E. (1994). *Creative scripts for hypnotherapy.* New York: Brunner Mazel.

James, F.R., Large, R.G., & Beale, I.L. (1989). Self-Hypnosis in chronic pain: A multiple baseline study of five highly hypnotizable subjects. *Clinical Journal of Pain, 5,* 161–168.

Kearns, R.D., Turk, D.C., & Rudy, T. E. (1985). The West Haven-Yale Multidimensional Pain Inventory (WHYMP). *Pain, 23,* 345–356.

Knox, V.J., Gekoski, W.L., Shum, K., & McLaughlin, D.M. (1981). Analgesia for experimentally induced pain: Multiple sessions of acupuncture compared to hypnosis in high- and low-susceptible subjects. *Journal of Abnormal Psychology, 90,* 28–34.

Large, (1994). *Hypnosis for chronic pain: A critical review.* Paper presented at the 13th International Congress of Hypnosis, Melbourne, Australia, August, 1994.

Lasagna, L., Mosteller, F., von Felsinger, J.M., & Beecher, H. (1954). A study of the placebo response. *American Journal of Medicine, 16,* 770–779.

McCauley, J.D., Thelen, M.H., Frank, R.G., Willard, R.R., & Callen, K.E. (1983). Hypnosis compared to relaxation in the outpatient management of low back pain. *Archives of Physical Medicine Rehabilitation, 64,* 548–552.

McGlashan, T.H., Evans, F.J., & Orne, M.T. (1969). The nature of hypnotic analgesia and the placebo response to experimental pain. *Psychosomatic Medicine, 31,* 227–246.

Meichenbaum, D.H. (1977). *Cognitive-behavior modification: An integrative approach.* New York: Plenum Press.

Melzack, R. V. (1975). The McGill Pain Questionnaire: Major properties & scoring methods. *Pain,* 217–299.

Melzack, R., & Perry, C. (1975). Self-regulation of pain: the use of alpha-feedback and hypnotic training for the control of chronic pain. *Experimental Neurology, 46,* 452–469.

Miller, M.E., & Bowers, K.S. (1986). Hypnotic analgesia and stress inoculation in the reduction of pain. *Journal of Abnormal Psychology, 95,* 6–14.

National Institutes of Mental Health Technology Assessment Conference. (1995). Integration of behavioral and relaxation approaches into the treatment of chronic pain and insomnia. Bethesda, Maryland, press release, October 5, 1995.

Olness, K., MacDonald, J.T., & Uden, D.L. (1987). Comparison of self-hypnosis and propranolol in the treatment of juvenile classic migraine. *Pediatrics, 79,* 593–597.

Orne, M.T. (1974). Pain suppression by hypnosis and related phenomena. In J.J. Bonica (Ed.), *Pain.* New York: Raven Press.

Patterson, D.R., Adcock, R.J., Bombadier, G. H. (1997). Factor predicting hypnotic analgesia in clinical burn patients. *International Journal of Clinical and Experimental Hypnosis, 45,* 377–395.

Prior, A., Colgan, S.M., & Whorwell, P.J. (1990). Changes in rectal sensitivity after hypnotherapy in patients with irritable bowel syndrome. *Gut, 31,* 896–898.

Rudy, T.E. (1989). *Multiaxial assessment of pain: Multidimensional pain inventory. Computer program users manual. Version 2.1. Technical report.* Pain Evaluation and Treatment Unit, Pittsburgh, PA.

Sacerdote, P. (1970). Theory and practice of pain control in malignancy and other protracted or recurring painful illnesses. *International Journal of Clinical and Experimental Hypnosis, 18,* 160–180.

Sarbin, T.R., & Coe, W. (1972). *Hypnosis: A social psychological analysis of influence communication.* New York: Holt, Rinehart & Winston.

Shor, R.E. (1962). Physiological effects of painful stimulation during hypnotic analgesia under conditions designed to minimize anxiety. *International Journal of Clinical and Experimental Hypnosis, 10,* 183–202.

Spanos, N.P. (1986). A social psychological approach to hypnotic behavior. *Behavior and Brain Sciences, 9,* 449–467.

Spiegel, D., & Albert, L.H. (1983). Naloxone fails to reverse hypnotic alleviation of chronic pain. *Psychopharmacology, 81,* 140–143.

Spiegel, D. (1993). *Living beyond limits.* New York: Times Books.

Spinhoven, P., Linssen, A.C., VanDyck, R., & Zitman, F.G. (1992). Autogenic training and self-hypnosis in the control of tension headache. *General Hospital Psychiatry, 14,* 408–415.

Stam, H.J., McGrath, P.A., & Brooke, R.I. (1984). The effects of a cognitive-behavioral treatment program on temporomandibular pain and dysfunction syndrome. *Psychosomatic Medicine, 46,* 534–545.

Sternbach, R.A. (1968). *Pain: A psychophysiological analysis.* New York: Academic Press.

Sternbach, R.A. (Ed.) (1986). *The psychology of pain.* New York: Raven Press.

Syrjala, K.L., Cummings, C., & Donaldson, G.W. (1992). Hypnosis or cognitive behavioral training for the reduction of pain and nausea during cancer treatment: A controlled clinical trial. *Pain, 48,* 137–146.

Tan, L.T., Tan, M.Y-C, & Veith (1973). *Acupuncture therapy: Current Chinese practice.* Philadelphia: Temple University Press.

Turk, D.C., Meichenbaum, D., & Genest, M. (1983). *Pain and behavioral medicine: A cognitive-behavioral perspective.* New York: Guilford.

Turner, J.A., & Chapman, C.R. (1982). Psychological interventions for chronic pain: A critical review. II. Operant conditioning, hypnosis, and cognitive-behavioral therapy. *Pain, 12,* 23–46.

Unestahl, L.E. (1979). Hypnotic preparation of athletes. In G.D. Burrows, D.R. Collison, & L. Dennerstein. *Hypnosis.* New York: Elsevier.

VanDyck, R., Zitman, F.G., Linssen, A.C., & Spinhoven, P. (1991). Autogenic training and future oriented imagery in the treatment of tension headache: Outcome and process. *International Journal of Clinical and Experimental Hypnosis, 39,* 6–23.

Wagstaff, G.F. (1981). *Hypnosis, compliance and belief.* New York: St. Martin's Press.

Wagstaff, G.F. (1987). Is hypnotherapy a placebo? *British Journal of Experimental and Clinical Hypnosis, 4,* 135–140.

Whorwill, P.J., Prior, A., and Faragher, E.B. (1984). Controlled trial of hypnotherapy in the treatment of severe refractory irritable-bowel syndrome. *Lancet,* 1232–1234.

Zitman, F.G., vanDyck, R., Spinhoven, P., & Linssen, A.C. (1992). Hypnosis and autogenic training in the treatment of tension headaches: A two phase constructive design study with follow-up. *Journal of Psychosomatic Research, 36,* 219–228.

Chapter 3

HYPNOSIS IN CONJUNCTION WITH CHEMICAL ANESTHESIA

LILLIAN E. FREDERICKS

GENERAL OBSERVATIONS

It is a well-established fact that almost all patients experience a great deal of anxiety and additional stress prior to surgery, especially when general anesthesia with the loss of consciousness has been suggested by the surgeon or the anesthesiologist. Some patients express great concern about the loss of control and the feelings which they experienced during previous anesthesias as well as negative encounters with doctors, dentists, and hospitals in general. It is important to find out what happened in previous experiences, relating to anesthesia and surgery, in order to reframe their perceptions of their experience and eliminate their fears and concerns. Even when patients need to go to a laboratory for tests or to a hospital for x rays or for an MRI, they experience heightened anxiety and stress (Quirk, Letendre, Ciottone & Lingley, 1989). Suddenly they are confronted with the possibility of a major illness, pain, or the necessity for surgery. All this, but especially surgery constitutes a major psychological stress (Kolough, 1968; Spielberger, 1973; Salmon, 1992). It is of interest to note that Weinberger, Gold and Sternberg (1984) showed that epinephrine fixes memory and it has been shown that fear, anxiety, and any kind of trauma releases epinephrine. We also know that anxiety influences the physical reaction to the stress of anesthesia and surgery. The preoperative psychological state of patients will also have a decided influence upon their recovery. Patients under high stress experience more pain, need more sedation, are prone to infections, show delayed healing (Rossi & Cheek, 1988, p. 360), and in general show a poor and prolonged recovery (Johnston, 1980; Ridgeway & Mathews, 1982), and Sime (1976) showed the least favorable recovery is associated with high levels of preoperative fear. Pert (1997, p. 188) has shown that the neuropeptides (the information molecules) and their specific receptors are not only in the brain, but are distributed throughout the body. They are the messengers carrying information to link all systems of the body into one unit, which she calls the body-mind. We have to think of it as a unit, not to be separated and having a reciprocal relationship. It has been known for centuries that the mind can influence the body, but now we know that it is not only the brain, with its peptides and specific receptors, sending messages to various parts of the body. Peptides and their receptors are found abundantly in the autonomic nervous system, regulating functions we previously thought were beyond our control and regulated only by the neurotransmitters, norepinephrine, and acetylcholine.

The anxiety may be due to uncertainty, threat of disability, deformity or death, economic loss, or to a combination of some or all of the above mentioned. Patients' reaction to stress depends upon the way they perceive the threat and the perception depends upon individual and cultural pressures, previous experiences, and the perceived meaning of the threat. Inappropriate responses to this increased stress may have detrimental consequences, as evidenced by derangements of various physiological functions. Emotions and feelings, both negative as well as positive, exert a direct influence on various physiological functions. The conscious and unconscious parts of our mind work in unison with our body. Each reacts instantaneously to the other.

Critically ill, disoriented, hemorrhaging, or severely injured patients go into a state of altered consciousness which is analogous to hypnosis. Bernheim was the first to show that "very sick and unconscious people behave as though hypnotized," cited in Yapko (1996). Rossi and Cheek (1988, p. 186) state, "The critically ill are already in a state of hypnosis." They enter a hypnotic state spontaneously. The same is true of patients being admitted to a hospital for major surgery (Cheek, 1962a; Rossi & Cheek, 1988, p. 131). They concentrate intensely on the caregiver, whether a physician or a nurse. They exclude their surroundings, take words literally, in a child-like manner (Erickson, 1980; Rossi & Cheek, 1988, p. 179) and often misinterpret comments made by persons of authority, such as physicians, technicians, or even friends and members of their own family. It seems that conscious, critical thinking is suspended and replaced by a phylogenetically older, more primitive way of thinking, a primary process thinking. Patients seem to be emotionally regressed. In this condition, they become very suggestible, and practitioners of the healing arts need to recognize and utilize this to the advantage of their patients. It is important to protect them because in this state, innocuous words, sentences, or careless conversations can be misinterpreted and may have detrimental effects (Cheek, 1960). This state of altered awareness (spontaneously occurring hypnosis) is a naturally occurring defense mechanism. It appears spontaneously when humans are frightened, disoriented, or in situations of severe violent stress, either mental or physical and quite possibly even when unconsciousness is physically or chemically induced.

There is overwhelming evidence and a vast body of literature documenting that patients perceive and encode meaningful information, even when in deep planes of surgical anesthesia (Pearson, 1961). Brunn (1963) reported from personal experience and Kihlstrom, Evans, Orne, and Orne (1980) state, "Information processing goes on in sleep and anesthesia." Enqvist (1996, p. 81) states that "implicit (indirect) memory of information given during general anesthesia has been shown, as well as improved recovery, after therapeutic suggestions given during general anesthesia." Levinson (1965) reported that when during surgery, upon a prearranged signal by the anesthesiologist, the surgeon suddenly, in a much disturbed voice said: "Is the patient all right? His blood is awfully dark!" the patient's pulse rate markedly increased and her blood pressure fell precipitously, even though nothing was changed outwardly. Experiences like these are not uncommon and one can witness the same kind of response when the diagnosis of a malignancy is announced over the intercom. The patient's blood pressure may go up or down precipitously, even at a time when there is no change in anesthesia or surgical stimulation.

Postoperative questioning for memories such as "Did you hear anything during your surgery" yields only negative results. There is dense amnesia. This amnesia has been shown to be a real inability to remember and a genuine forgetting. The forgotten material is stored in the brain but not available to the conscious mind (Kihlstrom & Schachter, 1990). However, when hypnotized and regressed to the operative experience and ideomotor finger signals are used, one can get a great deal of information about what the patient heard or perceived. Surgical anesthesia apparently blocks conscious, declarative verbal memory. When hypnotized and accessed on a nonverbal, behavioral level, such as pulling on an ear, verbal memories are accessed by ideomotor signaling (Bennett, Davis & Gianini, 1985). Consciousness is not necessary for hearing and imprinting memory. Words can be perceived and cause a response on an unconscious level without conscious awareness. There is unconscious encoding of meaningful sensory perceptual information constantly, not only under surgical anesthesia, but also in comatose and critically ill patients. Bonke, Fitsh, and Miller (1990) published a book on awareness under anesthesia. Munglani and Jones (1994) report that information processing and implicit memory during general anesthesia are real phenomena and can occur even during adequate chemical anesthesia. Wolfe and Millet (1960) decreased postoperative pain by suggestions made under general anesthesia. Bonke, Smitz, Verhage, and Zwaveling (1986) were able to reduce hospital stay in elderly patients with the use of positive suggestions during surgery. Evans and Richardson (1988) reported improved recovery and reduced hospital stay following suggestions given during general anesthesia. McLintock, Aitken, Downie, and Kenny (1990) also showed that intraoperative suggestions decrease the amount of morphine postoperatively for the control of pain. Dillon, Minchoff, and Baker (1985) state that the endocrine and immune systems react positively or negatively to suggestions made during surgery. Olness, Culbert, and Uden (1989) reported changes in salivary immunoglobulin A in children using hypnosis, and Black (1994) showed that IgA levels were significantly increased in subjects who underwent a hypnotic induction prior to being exposed to a stressor.

The unconscious interprets in a literal, childlike manner, whether patients are conscious or unconscious. Reassurance often is accepted on a conscious level, but may be rejected by the unconscious. However, indirect assurance is always accepted at an unconscious level. For example, if we say to a patient, "You will have no postoperative pain or complications" and give good reasons for it, the patient may accept this on a conscious, thinking level, but his or her unconscious may reject this and expect pain and some postoperative complications. When talking to patients about all the activities in which they will partake the day after surgery and how they will enjoy the food and their company, they will unconsciously accept the fact that they will do well. This is an example of indirect assurance. At the same time, patients will also lose their unconscious fear of death, because indirect suggestions of lack of complications and the enjoyment of tender loving care which they will experience made them accept the premise that they will have survived the operation.

Here are some examples to show how patients perceive and imprint during surgical anesthesia and often interpret in a literal, childlike manner. In the operating room, one frequently hears a surgeon say, "Let's get out of here and go home," meaning to get out of the abdomen and close the abdominal wall. The patient may perceive this as being abandoned by the surgeon and turned over to an assistant. Or "She will never be the same" said to a patient who underwent the removal of a gangrenous gallbladder. The surgeon wanted to say that she is better off without her gallbladder, but the patient misinterpreted it to mean that she will be a different person. She liked the way she was and did not want to be different. Postoperatively she became extremely angry at the surgeon and did not want to see him ever again, even though she was not aware of the reason. Cheek (1965) discussed the sequel occurring postoperatively in patients who perceived important communications intraoperatively.

There are a few sentences which need to be stricken from our vocabulary when dealing with patients in the operating room such as: "Now I will put you to sleep," meaning I will now administer the anesthetic. The patient in childhood may have lost a pet, which was "put to sleep" by a kind veterinarian, an experience which might have been quite traumatic and stored in the subconscious. It also may be very frightening to patients when emerging from anesthesia to hear the anesthesiologist proclaim, "You are finished," or "it's all over." Or if the patient wakes up while the surgeon puts in the last few stitches, "Hold still, it will be all over in a few minutes." These and many other statements made by persons of authority may be misinterpreted by patients and may lead to drastic changes in their psychological and physical condition.

The avoidance of psychological trauma is very important. It may occur not only during surgery, but also at any time during the hospital stay. Patients are very vulnerable to indirect suggestions and to misinterpretations of conversations they might overhear, or suggestions which are made directly to them. Patients even respond unconsciously to the way in which persons of authority answer their questions. For instance, patients may ask about their recovery period and the length of time they will need to remain in the hospital. If the surgeon answers "5 or 10 days," that is an indirect suggestion that there may be some complications and that the patient will need to stay in the hospital a longer period of time than is usually required. An example of a direct suggestion is the following. A well-known anesthesiologist gave several thousands spinal anesthetics for transurethral resection of the prostate gland while in an army hospital and saw very few spinal headaches (1%–2% which is the accepted risk). After the war, when working in a university hospital, the incidence of postspinal headaches was about 80 percent. He frantically searched for the cause of this dramatic difference and luckily, one day he overheard the urologist say to one of his patients, "Don't let them give you a spinal, you will get an awful headache." The surgeon had programmed all his patients with a direct suggestion, while they were in a state of heightened awareness and increased suggestibility, and no matter how the anesthesiologist explained the advantages and the comfort of spinal anesthesia, even though these patients accepted this on a logical, conscious level, unconsciously they were programmed to get an awful headache and it made no difference what the anesthesiologist said; they developed an awful headache (personal communication).

Using hypnosis postoperatively, it is possible to elicit verbatim recitals of important intraoperative events. Ewin (1994) states that implicit memory can be accessed in hypnosis, recovering details of a trauma not available in explicit memory. My first and most dramatic experience with this phenomenon was when I heard a surgeon scream at the top of his voice, "Isn't anybody going to help me? Are you going to let this patient bleed to death?" He said this to his assistants during open heart surgery, when with finger rupture of the mitral valve severe hemorrhage occurred, and the surgeon could not see the origin of the severed vessel. The patient's blood pressure dropped, her pulse rate increased, and we had to replace the large amount of blood she lost, which had not been anticipated prior to surgery. I immediately bent down to the patient's ear, addressed her by her first name, assured her that all was under control, that her vital signs were stable, that the surgery was progressing well, and that she should continue to be as comfortable and relaxed as she was before. The patient had no ill effects and no adverse reaction to this frightening experience. In all likelihood, this was due to the intervention, namely the immediate communication and reassurance I gave her during anesthetic unconsciousness. She was prepared preoperatively with hypnotic techniques and knew that I would be able to communicate with her, even at a time when she was sufficiently anesthetized, unconscious and completely free of any discomfort. I saw her postoperatively in the intensive care unit and also the following morning. She expressed her gratitude and said that she was surprised that the surgery took such a short time. This is the result of time distortion, which is a phenomenon typical of hypnosis. She did not recall anything unusual. I got her permission to use hypnosis and after a rapid induction I took her through the operative experience. She nicely went through the induction of anesthesia and remarked on the vivid imagery she experienced apparently for just a little while and then she fell silent. At one point, she became quite apprehensive and asked me what is going on? I gave her time to relive this particular event. I then explained ideomotor finger signals to her (Cheek, 1962b) mentioning that often the subconscious knows more about a situation than the conscious mind (Yapko, 1990), and I asked her permission whether it would be all right to remember and talk about what she heard or perceived at that time. Her yes finger responded and after a few moments, she quoted verbatim the entire tirade of the surgeon. This to me was the most amazing experience. It is known that on occasions patients can perceive meaningful information, even in deep planes of general anesthesia, but I did not know that it could be as accurate a replay as this patient was able to transmit to me. David Cheek had a large sign in his operating room which read "Your patient is listening to you" (personal communication). Ewin (1994) states that "in humans, implicit memory can be accessed in hypnosis, recovering details of a trauma not available in explicit memory."

To allay the anxiety and the tremendous stress put upon the patient, the doctor-patient relationship should be such that the patient perceives the surgeon and the anesthesiologist as allies. The patient must be educated to have a realistic image of the surgical experience. The entire hospital stay and especially the surgical procedure can be made much more comfortable and tolerable by paying attention not only to the physical, but also to the emotional and mental state of patients. The anesthesiologist plays an important role in decreasing the added stress and anxiety. Surgeons often are too busy to devote time to develop an interpersonal relationship with their patients. Anesthesiologists have a specific time set aside, namely the preoperative visit or interview, to explain procedures and answer questions in an unhurried manner. In doing so they create trust and confidence and also help patients to gain a realistic picture of the surgical and anesthesia experience (Rodger, 1961; Fredericks, 1978). Egbert, Battit, and Turndorf (1963) showed that a five-minute visit decreases preoperative anxiety, postoperative pain, and the use of analgesics. Evans and Stanley (1991) reviewed the literature and found several hypnotic techniques which could be used successfully prior to surgery.

Various kinds of psychological interventions, including the teaching of auto-hypnosis, have shown reductions of postoperative psychosis (Lazarus & Hagens, 1968), time spent in the intensive care unit (Fortin & Kirouac, 1976), intubation time (Surman, Hacket & Behrendt 1974), length of hospitalization (Rogers & Reich 1986), postoperative vomiting (Dumas & Leonard 1963), as well as the need for catheterization. Goldman, Ogg, and Levey (1988) reported earlier discharges from the hospital, as well as the need for fewer medications, the use of which might have caused complications. Enqvist and Ficher (1997) report a decrease in the use of analgesics following dental surgery and, Enqvist summarized the results of 5 studies using presurgical hypnosis as well as suggestions under general anesthesia. Hypnotically prepared patients have a much smoother and shorter convalescence (Pearson, 1961; Egbert, Battit, Welsh & Bartlett, 1964). The mechanisms of healing, the rapid recovery, and lack of complications can be intentionally mobilized by psychological interventions. There is also a direct relationship between specific suggestions and the effect on involuntary processes, such as blood loss during surgery (Bennett, Benson & Kuicken, 1985), visceral and glandular responses (Miller, 1969), and increase or decrease of gastric secretions (Klein & Spiegel, 1989). Mittleman, Doubt, and Gravitz (1992) showed a faster rate of heat loss when subjects were told to feel warm.[1] Houghton, Heyman, and Whorwell (1996) treated irritable bowel syndrome with hypnosis, not only relieving the symptoms successfully, but also showing improvement in the quality of life, and Casiglia et al. (1997) were able to achieve, with good hypnotic subjects, with appropriate suggestions of undergoing phlebotomy, the same changes in blood pressure and

---

1. The suggestion of feeling warm causes vaso dilatation in highly hypnotizable subjects leading to greater heat loss.

peripheral resistance as subjects who actually underwent phlebotomy.

Hypnosis and hypnotic techniques are excellent tools for the proper preparation of patients for major surgery, or any other painful or anxiety provoking medical or surgical intervention. Zimmerman (1998) has successfully used this technique in 200 patients undergoing upper gastrointestinal endoscopy. Patients who experience a relatively low level of anxiety go into trance readily, when spoken to as if a formal induction had just been completed. Patients in high stress are often in a state of altered awareness and high suggestibility, but they will listen only when their imagination is caught with vivid imagery and relevant communication. Erickson (1982), with his "Hint and Run" technique, has taught us to turn a negative, dismal view into a positive attitude through vivid imagery. With proper suggestions, the mind can quickly paint a very real and pleasant picture to bypass a destructive, negative attitude and replace it with a positive one. Hypnosis can distort reality perception, memory, and mood in response to appropriate suggestions. A flow of carefully worded suggestions telling the patient what to expect and how to react comfortably, presented in a low and confident voice will reassure them. When making these suggestions and gradually lowering our voice and gradually drifting into a slow and rhythmic manner of speech, making appropriate pauses to allow the patient to follow our suggestions carefully, patients will usually deepen their trance or slip into it if they were not in hypnosis before.

It is important to ascertain the coping style of each particular patient. Patients need to be informed about what will be done to physically prepare them for the induction of anesthesia and all the various procedures which will precede it. Some patients repress all their emotions and detailed explanations would only increase their anxiety (Auerbach, 1989). On the other hand, some patients, the vigilant ones, need to be informed, on their level of understanding. Explanations about the surgery and some details about the anesthesia will help them to cope with situations, which otherwise might be frightening and overwhelming to them. Kessler (1997) summarized this in an excellent article, pointing out the importance of evaluating the coping style of each patient and thereby selecting the proper clinical strategies. This can be done easily by just asking the patient "would you like to know more about your anesthesia and surgery?"[2]

---

2. Vigilant patients will want to be informed in great detail, but avoidant patients often will say "I don't want to know anything, just put me to sleep"

Hypnotizability, does not play an important role in the context of anxiety reduction (Schoenberger quoted by Kirsch, 1994). Barber (1993) observed that a high score does not guarantee clinical efficacy, and low hypnotizability does not guarantee clinical inefficacy, and Barber (1996) discusses hypnotic analgesia and reaffirms that hypnotic scales are less useful in clinical situations than in laboratory settings. Hypnotizability is fairly stable in each individual patient and the largest proportion of the population scores in the medium or low range. This group of patients should not be deprived of the advantages hypnosis and hypnotic techniques would give them. Interestingly, Houge (1997) reported that among ten consecutive patients undergoing surgery with hypnosis as the sole anesthetic, none of them tested as "high hypnotizable" (Stanford Form C). Had he discouraged these ten patients from using hypno-anesthesia, he would have deprived them from the safest method of anesthesia and from a very interesting and gratifying experience. When taking care of patients, both in the operating room, as well as in the emergency room, short procedure area, radiology department, etc., it is not necessary to test for hypnotic capacity in a formal way. It might have a negative effect and would waste precious time. However, Greenleaf, Fisher, Miaskowski, and DuHamel (1992) found that hypnotic capacity is a good predictor of postoperative recovery in patients undergoing heart surgery. When doing clinical research, it is mandatory to test for hypnotic capacity, but this also takes risks, decreasing the effectiveness of therapeutic suggestions, in case the patient tests poorly and fails several items on the scales.

The depth of trance during these interventions is not important either. For instance, glove anesthesia can be produced in relatively light planes of hypnosis. Patients unconsciously seek the level necessary to follow suggestions given by their caregiver in order to achieve their goal. Nevertheless, when necessary, deepening techniques such as imagining ocean waves, waterfalls, going down steps, etc., need to be used to deepen trance. It is very important to choose techniques that are relevant and appropriate for each individual patient.

Frequently, physicians say, "It takes too much additional time to use hypnosis." As a rule, this is not true. In fact, it takes less time when dealing with a patient who is uncooperative or completely stressed out (Fredericks, 1980). Under these circumstances, it takes less time to achieve a specific goal, because with the use of hypnosis, patients accept our suggestions uncritically, become relaxed, confident, and cooperate with us. Pearson (1973) states that almost all patients can achieve some level of trance. Therefore, one should offer hypnosis or hypnotic techniques to all surgical patients. As a rule, they are under considerable emotional stress, quite motivated and receptive to positive suggestions.

There is no need for a formal induction of hypnosis because patients in such situations are already in a state of altered awareness (Rossi & Cheek 1988, p 186) and are very suggestible and one can proceed as though trance had been induced. Therefore, special mention of the use of hypnosis on an informed consent document, which the patient must sign prior to surgery, will not be necessary. Hypnotic sequelae in clinical practice, in connection with surgery, are extremely rare. Coe, Peterson, and Gwynn (1995) stated that patients with whom possible ill effects were discussed showed a greater number of sequelae. Thus, it seems contraindicated to mention complications. It is possible that mentioning ill effects, in general, may act like unintended suggestions, which are accepted because of the increased suggestibility of patients.

Hypnotic techniques should be used routinely as part of caring for patients as an anesthesiologist. Bartlett (1966) pointed out that hypnotic techniques utilize normal, simple, natural methods to modify or control inappropriate behavior by suggestions, without the formal induction of hypnosis. Hypnotic techniques are uniquely suitable for any patient's needs at any time of temporary stress. To a great extent these techniques use subcortical communication, which is an appeal to the emotional side of the brain, rather than neocortical communication which appeals to reason and logic. She pointed out that this subcortical communication is a psychological language, which is largely nonverbal. It uses images, feelings, symbols, and metaphors. Words are translated into feelings, images, and symbols spontaneously by the patient. These suggestions must invite patients to create and produce those feelings and moods which are comforting and reassuring to them. To teach patients and communicate with them in such a way, will lead to the acceptance of the suggestions. She suggests that we should speak with a soft, confident, reassuring voice, making only positive suggestions, and to choose our words carefully to avoid misinterpretations by the patient (Bartlett, 1971).

Using hypnotic techniques, making specific, positive, and appropriate suggestions during the preoperative visit, during induction of anesthesia as well as during surgery and postoperatively, patients will have a smooth recovery, less pulmonary problems, faster wound healing, fewer infections, less need for narcotics, and a shorter hospital stay than patients who were not prepared with hypnotic techniques. Magaw (1906) was a well-known anesthesiologist at the Mayo Clinic who used suggestions and who talked patients to sleep with as little ether as possible. She reported 14,000 consecutive anesthesias without a death. Among others, Bensen (1971), Ewin (1984), Fredericks (1988), and Rossi and Cheek (1990) have been routinely using these techniques of preparing patients with psychological interventions. Field (1974) also prepared patients with hypnosis prior to surgery, but used commercial tapes rather than adapting the procedure to each individual patient.

Preparation of the Patient

During the routine preoperative visit, one should evaluate quickly the degree of the patient's apprehension. After the introduction, it is important to shake the patient's hand, noticing the temperature, the dryness or moisture, the muscle tension or relaxation of the hand. Taking the patient's pulse, keeping the hand on the patient's hand should be routine. This bodily contact establishes rapport quickly. There is a great deal of extra verbal communication through the human touch. Pert (1997, p. 272), from her own experience, states, "I know the power of touch to stimulate and regulate our natural chemicals, the ones that are tailored to act at precisely the right times in exactly the appropriate dosages to maximize our feelings of health and well-being." To notice the color of the patient's face, its expression, the presence of perspiration, all are meaningful. It is mandatory to observe patients very carefully and when a question is not immediately answered, to watch to which side the patient's gaze is directed. There is a relationship between hypnotic capacity and the direction of the gaze. It has been shown that good hypnotic subjects gaze to the left and medium or lows gaze to the right. Duke (1968) reported that 86 percent of subjects were consistent in the direction of eye movements and Bakan (1969, p. 929) found that "13 of the 18 right-movers fell into the low hypnotizibility group, and 16 of 24 left-movers fell into the high hypnotizibility group." Sitting down leisurely rather than towering over the patient invites a pleasant atmosphere. It is important to state the purpose of the visit, to ascertain what the patient likes, as well as any strong dislikes or phobias. Patients need assurance that the anesthesiologist is familiar with their condition and with the contemplated surgery "which will take care of your problem." This in itself is an indirect suggestion that surgery will be successful and that they will be well thereafter.

Patients need to be taught to relax in a very special way, a way which they have never experienced before. It is good to ask the patient, "Where would you like to be right now, rather than here in this hospital?" Patients find another place with the greatest of ease. Their response will indicate where patients will be in their mind's eye, when in hypnosis and dissociated to this pleasant place of their choice. It is extremely important to help patients to dissociate from the operating room. They can leave their body on the operating table to be taken care of, but transport their feelings and emotions to a different place, where they can be comfortable and safe.

Following this, one might say, "Would you like me to show you a way to go through tomorrow's anesthesia and surgery with comfort and safety?" All patients accept this with pleasure. Patients want to be comfortable and safe. At this time, eye closure might be suggested and the taking of a deep breath and "as you exhale let all your muscles go limp and loose and relaxed from the top of your head all the way down to the tip of your toes." This method of inducing relaxation seems to be much more successful than starting from the feet and working up to the head, a technique which has been taught repeatedly. Relaxation is a downward movement. To tell patients, who are stressed to the limit, to take it easy and to relax is ineffective. Patients would relax if they could, because stress is extremely uncomfortable. One needs to teach patients to relax by appropriate suggestions such as " go limp and loose like a rag doll, or like a wet flag hanging down when there is no wind," etc. It is best not to mention the word "hypnosis." It would necessitate spending time with lengthy explanations about hypnosis, clearing up all misconceptions and preventing any resistance which might occur when talking about hypnosis.

When helping patients to dissociate to a place of their choice and encouraging them to observe all the details of the place, one might suggest to "see all the beautiful and interesting things, hear familiar sounds, touch some of the objects, really feel that you are there, and thoroughly enjoy every minute." It is important for the professional to be relaxed as well, to be truly involved and in no hurry. Patients are very perceptive and react to their impressions. When trying to be a role model and be relaxed and comfortable, it is possible to slip into trance oneself, which is in no way contraindicated. What better way to serve patients than to intently concentrate upon them, excluding the surroundings and paying attention only to the subject at hand. When it becomes obvious that patients are following these positive suggestions, the next important part of the intervention can begin, namely the giving of suggestions, which will teach them to help their bodies to accomplish specific goals.

Suggestions

Observations of several well-known clinicians such as Cheek (1962a) and Rossi and Cheek (1988, p. 131) that surgical patients are in a state of altered awareness and increased suggestibility necessitates the very careful choice of words and concentration on making appropriate suggestions. In general, only positive suggestions should be made to influence the behavior of patients, because they are more readily accepted than negative suggestions. The relationship between the patient and the clinician is of paramount importance. Patients perceive competence or the lack of it, and hopefully confidence and trust will follow. Instructions become suggestions. Peter B. Burkhard (1998, p. 68) said that an instruction becomes a suggestion when it is "so obviously right and proper that it doesn't even enter one's head not to obey it." Words are like drugs, especially when they are accompanied by warm, compassionate, and sincere feelings. Suggestions should foster hope, positive expectations, understanding, and empathy. One should try to give a good reason why patients should accept them and what they can expect to achieve by following them. Suggestions need to be highly idiosyncratic and in response to each patient's needs and expectations. Thoughtful attention needs to be given to the required informed consent. The more complications are mentioned, the more likely it is that patients will develop them. We try not to go into any details of what can happen, but rather assure patients that with today's new anesthetic agents and techniques and with the kind of preparation they are receiving at this time, they will do very well and they will be pleasantly surprised how quickly the time passed and how much more comfortable they were than they expected to be. There is a need to prepare patients for the unexpected by assuring them that their bodies are capable of shifting gears easily and without problems, in case surgery has to be modified.

When suggestions are accepted by patients, praise is in order. "That's good, that's very good." Praise is very important when using hypnotic techniques. Patients do not know what to do, how to proceed, what to expect and how to follow suggestions and they need to be told when they are successful. Repetition is also important. Even individual words need to be repeated several times, such as "deeper and deeper and deeper, and more and more comfortable," etc.

At times, it is appropriate to explain to patients what will be done to prepare them for a safe, comfortable, and relaxed anesthesia, "so the surgeon can do the proposed operation to the best of his or her ability." The assurance that we will be with them the entire time watching their blood pressure, heart rate, and all other vital functions is very comforting to them. The fact that we will be able to communicate with them, even though they are deeply anesthetized and comfortable, needs to be presented in a delicate and caring way. It is very interesting to see that a statement like this does not seem to frighten patients, provided it is delivered appropriately. At this time, patients feel comfortable and safe with their caregivers and they know intuitively that they would not misinform them, or harm them in any way. With the use of hypnosis, a very intense interpersonal relationship is formed and there develops a great deal of transference and countertransference. To say, "you will be free of pain," might subconsciously lead to misinterpretations. The word pain should not be used at any time, because it may conjure up some very powerful and disturbing memories. "You will be comfortable and relaxed" are proper suggestions.

It has been shown that even in deep surgical anesthesia, patients are able to perceive meaningful information. David Cheek, as early as 1959, observed and reported unconscious perception of meaningful sounds during surgical anesthesia, and gave a detailed report in 1964. Breckenridge and Aitkenhead (1983) reviewed the literature up to that time and later, Rossi and Cheek (1988, p. 113) stated that "meaningful sounds, meaningful silence, meaningful conversation are registered and may have a profound influence upon behavior of the patient, during surgery and for many years after." Jones and Konieczko (1986); McLintock, Aitken, Downie, and Kenny (1990); Evans and Richardson (1988); Pearson (1961); Mark and Greenberg (1983); and Howard (1987) all report similar observations. Because of this, patients are told they need to pay attention only to the voice of their anesthesiologist or surgeon and only when addressed by name. To hear the sound of that voice even without listening, all the other sounds seem far away, just like background music and nothing will disturb them. It is amazing how noisy most operating rooms are, with nurses preparing instruments and frequently dropping some, with their never-ending conversations of what they did last night, what TV they watched, or what movie they saw, loudspeakers paging physicians and so on. Being exposed to these noises every day for years, one gets accustomed to them and can ignore them completely. However, they are very disturbing to a patient who is unfamiliar with the routine of an operating room. A nice way is to tell patients that all these noises are the result of the nurses getting ready for the surgery, preparing everything which the surgeon may need. Treating anesthetized patients as though they were conscious is very important (Rossi and Cheek, 1988, p. 131). There should not be much difference in the way one talks to anesthetized patients and those under local or regional anesthesia.

Patients need to be informed that they can help their bodies to bleed very little during surgery, by constricting their tiny little bloodvessels and by shunting the blood away from the operative site to other parts of their body. Grabowska (1971) showed that subjects under hypnosis and with pertinent suggestions were able to influence their blood flow. "Thoughts of coldness can constrict blood vessels" (Rossi & Cheek, 1988 p. 193). Chaves (1980) and Bishay, Stevens, and Lee (1984) controlled an upper gastrointestinal hemorrhage with the use of hypnosis, and Bennet, Benson, and Kuiken (1986) were able to show in a well-controlled study, measuring blood loss during spine surgery, a significant decrease in bleeding with patients who were given preoperative instructions to help their bodies to control bleeding. Among others, Enqvist, Konow, and Bystedt (1995) achieved a 30 percent reduction in blood loss during maxillofacial surgery, making appropriate suggestions preoperatively. Moore and Wiesner (1996) showed that patients can shift blood to a predetermined part of their body, such as a hand, via vasodilatation and, in doing so, they were able to increase the temperature by an average of 6.71 degrees Fahrenheit. It is astonishing what patients can accomplish with the use of hypnosis, which makes them aware of the enormous power of their unconscious mind. With patients suffering from hemophilia, bleeding can be stopped even in massive hemorrhage which might occur spontaneously or due to surgery. Rasputin, the Russian monk (1871-1916), supposedly was able to stop bleeding in the Czarevitch by putting him in a trance using hypnosis. Lucas (1965) used hypnosis to control bleeding occurring during a tooth extraction and, in 1975, he published his use of hypnosis in dental care of hemophiliacs. Fredericks (1967) stopped bleeding in a hemophiliac following a gastrectomy and LaBaw (1975) taught children self-hypnosis to control their bleeding. Dubin and Shapiro (1977) reported using hypnosis in a hemophiliac to stop bleeding due to dental extraction. Swersky-Saechetti and Margolis (1986) studied the use of factor VIII in patients with severe hemophilia and showed that when using self-hypnosis there was much less need for blood replacement.

It is most important to inform the patient that upon awakening from anesthesia, he or she might find the presence of various devices such as a naso-gastric catheter, a catheter in her or his bladder, an endotracheal tube in her or his mouth, etc. and the reason why they are there. This is mandatory when there is the possibility that the patient may remain on a respirator after surgery. It is very frightening to come out of anesthesia and not be able to breathe and not be able to speak, having an endotracheal tube in place. When patients have been informed of these possibilities and the purpose of each intervention has been explained, they are prepared and will not panic upon awakening. Patients will understand why they are having these otherwise frightening gadgets, since this was planned ahead and not because something went wrong.

At the end of surgery, patients should expect to wake up promptly and comfortably, feeling as though they just awakened from a good night's sleep, being happy and surprised that it was much easier and much shorter than they expected it to be (time distortion). Soon they will feel thirsty and hungry, looking forward to the next meal. This suggestion is made only if the type of surgery allows oral intake soon postoperatively. Otherwise, one may say, "you will feel hungry and thirsty" as soon as it is appropriate. This suggestion avoids nausea and vomiting. If one is thirsty and hungry, one cannot be nauseated. Any sensation which they might have in the operative area will tell them that healing has begun already. "Let this be a signal to you to let that area get limp and loose, soft and relaxed." Patients need to be informed that all the physiological functions will return promptly, such as urination and bowel movements. It will be easy to breathe deeply, cough, and clear their throats. Expectation on the part of the patient influences the outcome.

It is important to tell patients that, while they are in the hospital, they have "so much time" to enjoy the physical rest and the tender loving care which they will receive, they can enjoy their visitors and plan the return to their home. This guidance to look into the future and see how well they are doing, without the impediment created by the problem, which was corrected with surgery, indirectly helps them to realize that they will be alive and well again. Patients need to look forward only, and enjoy all the things which make life more productive, more interesting, and more enjoyable (Rossi & Cheek, 1988, p. 184). Torem (1992) beautifully describes such a technique, where he lets the patients decide what event in the future they want to witness, such as a wedding, a birthday party, or an outing with the family. He takes them to that point in time and encourages his patients to see images, hear sounds, touch and smell, and really feel that they are there. When encountering patients who have a tremendous fear of death, they usually will lose this fear when they concentrate on various things they will be able to do postoperatively, making plans for the future. However, if there is a patient, who after these suggestions outright says, "Doctor I am going to die during this operation," and there is no way to convince this patient that this does not have to be so, the surgery should be postponed, after consultation with the surgeon. Such a patient should be evaluated psychologically to find the cause for this extraordinary fear and be treated by a psychiatrist or psychologist before returning to surgery. Patients should be encouraged, with appropriate suggestions, to eradicate from their mind any pain or problems which they might have had prior to surgery. "Just like sailboats, always going forward, leaving the wake behind." There is nothing they can do to change the past, but there is so much they can do for today and in the future.

With the expectation of a sound and refreshing sleep the night prior to surgery, patients can look forward to meeting their surgeon and anesthesiologist in the operating room the following day. It is wise to give patients a choice whether they would like to be sedated prior to surgery or not. Vigilant patients usually prefer not to be sedated; they want to watch and know what is going on. However, there are patients whose mode of coping is avoidant, who would like to be asleep from the time they leave their room, even when they did well with the psychological preparation. When giving patients this choice, it adds to their feeling of being in control, which is very beneficial, rather than being just an object to be examined, tested, and operated upon.

Patients are encouraged to visualize their favorite scene and go to their place of comfort frequently, before and after surgery. This will relax them in a special way, and relaxed muscles heal faster, since there is no pull on them. If there is no pull, there is no pain. We also know that, when there is no pain, the chance of an infection is less, and healing is expedited due to increased blood flow to the affected area while thinking about warmth and comfort (Mishkin & Petri, 1984; Rossi & Cheek, 1988, p. 193).

In short, the suggestions and explanations of what will happen during anesthesia and surgery, what will be done to assure their safety and comfort, and what they can do to help their body to accomplish expected goals are the essence of the psychological preparation with hypnosis, which have been shown to change patients' expectations, attitudes, and psychological as well as physiological parameters. This not only will give patients a sense of competence and some measure of control, but it also will include them as active members of the team. These suggestions also encourage patients to concentrate intently on pleasant things, focus their attention and translate verbal suggestions into images and feelings and act upon them. This is not just loving, tender care, but giving very specific suggestions to achieve very specific goals. Erickson (1965) said so beautifully, "With the use of hypnosis and the semantics, that are an integral part of it, we strive to accomplish iatrogenic health by the use of words that heal." The use of hypnosis as a psychological intervention prior to surgery seems to have profound positive effects on many physiological parameters.

Body and mind have a reciprocal effect upon each other and they are inseparable. Our mind can have a very powerful influence upon our body. For example, Klein and Spiegel (1989) reported an increase or decrease of gastric acidity dependent upon suggestions and visual imagery. The immune system and T cell activity can be influenced with the use of appropriate suggestions during hypnosis. Smith, Barabasz, Barabasz, and Warner (1995) reported highly hypnotizable subjects exposed to hypnosis showed significant alterations of the immune system as measured by an increase of B-cells and T-cells. Johnson, Walker, Heys, Whiting, and Eremin (1996) showed that after three weeks of relaxation training, which was introduced by listening to an audio cassette of the Stanford Hypnotic Clinical Scale (Hilgard & Hilgard, 1983) and daily use of a relaxation tape and mental imagery, followed by a stressor, the experimental group showed IgA levels (measuring host defenses) significantly increased with relaxation. Followed by a stressor, they also obtained an increased lymphocyte response to PHA (mitogen response to Phytohaemagglutinin) and a significant increase in IL-1beta (Interleukin 1). On the third visit, experimental subjects were in much better spirits, more energetic, and clear-headed than control subjects. Olness (1997) trained 11 juveniles suffering from migraine headaches in self-hypnosis and reported a decrease in mast cell activation in nine of them, and Pert (1997) showed very convincingly the influence of emotions on our bodies, all of which confirms the impression that hypnosis, relaxation, and the concomitant uplifting emotions are beneficial to our health in many ways and that they strengthen the immune system, prevent infections, and promote general good health.

Observations

During this psychological preparation, patients relax visibly and often show definitive signs of being in an altered state of awareness. This can be recognized in many patients, by slowing down of respirations and pulse rate. Patients' facial expressions change, probably due to the complete relaxation of their facial musculature. They do not swallow and occasionally circumoral pallor can be observed. They are acutely aware and attentive to the meaning of suggestions as well as extraverbal communications such as touch.

When asked to leave their favorite place and open their eyes, they usually take a deep breath, rub their eyes, and stretch. A smile replaces the frown and anxious look on their faces, which were present prior to the hypnotic experience. Often, patients talk about the wonderful feelings they experienced during this session. By telling patients that they should practice going to their favorite place several times a day, they learn self-hypnosis and they realize that they can recreate these wonderful feelings and the refreshing relaxation all on their own. All they need to do is close their eyes, to eliminate visual distractions, visualize their favorite place, and thoroughly enjoy just being there. Using self-hypnosis can be formulated as a posthypnotic suggestion. It has been shown that patients remain hyper-suggestible for quite some time after they open their eyes and come out of trance. This is an appropriate time to tell them that when they use self-hypnosis they will notice that all the suggestions we gave them will be remembered, which will reinforce and anchor them in their unconscious mind. Patients should be encouraged to do this little exercise frequently for the rest of the day and on the way to the operating room, at which time someone will come with a stretcher to take them to the operating room.

Patients should be given the opportunity to ask questions and they should be answered as clearly as possible. Explanations need to be given on their level of understanding. It is interesting to see how pleased patients are at this point, perceiving that they found somebody who takes the time to listen to their questions and who helps them to better understand a very mysterious and frightening experience. Most people fear the unknown and are very grateful and relieved when they are given the opportunity to air their concerns.

It is good to meet patients in the holding area of the operating room suite, to greet them with a smile, and to inquire how they slept and how they feel right now. Invariably, patients are quite relaxed and really happy to see their friends again. Some patients are obviously in a state of altered consciousness, which they induced themselves.

After being accompanied into the operating room and helped to get on the table, patients often realize that what is being done for them is in their best interest and that no effort is spared. While preparing the patient for the induction of anesthesia, i.e., putting on the blood pressure cuff, checking the EKG, etc., it is appropriate to repeat the suggestions which were made the night before and explaining that all the noises around them are due to nurses preparing for the surgery, making sure that all is in perfect order and ready for the surgeon. "You need not pay any attention to this; it can be just like lovely, soft background music." If time permits, it is interesting for patients to let them look at the EKG monitor to show them how nicely and rhythmically their heart is beating. This makes patients involved and interested and prevents them from concentrating on frightening and disturbing thoughts. If patients are not sedated with the use of medications, it is important to engage them continuously during this time, because the unfamiliar surroundings of the operating room are anxiety provoking. If patients are sedated by their premedication, it is less important and it might be wise not to engage them in conversation at all. Even though the former are well relaxed and not anxious, it makes them feel good, and repetition in hypnosis is very important. During the preoperative visit, it is possible to develop a specific signal to go into hypnosis, such as a hand making pressure on their right shoulder or squeezing their right hand. This is a good time to use this. To suggest that patients go to their favorite place helps them to dissociate. They may leave their body here to be taken care of, but mentally go to their favorite place, involve all their senses, and really feel that they are there.

During the Induction of Anesthesia

Depending on the patient's coping mechanisms, vigilant patients need to be informed about all the procedures which need to be performed, prior to the actual induction of anesthesia, and also the reasons for executing them. When patients are of the avoidant type this will be omitted, since it would be counterproductive. Any additional information as far as anesthesia or surgery is concerned would greatly increase their anxiety. While starting the intravenous infusion, one may tell patients that the cool feeling from the antiseptic, which is used to cleanse the skin, will make the area "numb and pretty much asleep." When scrubbing the skin vigorously and flicking it with the fingernail a few times to make it numb, most patients do not even feel the insertion of the intravenous catheter, let alone feel pain. While connecting the various monitors and continuously talking to them in a soft and relaxed but confident voice, repeating many of the suggestions made previously, patients are mentally occupied, which prevents them from developing anxiety provoking thoughts. When the time comes to actually administer the anesthesia, the patient is usually well relaxed and busy with enjoying the place of their choice or mentally executing a favorite activity. During an intravenous induction with thiopenthal or any other medication, one might suggest, no matter where they are in their minds eye, it might be time to go to bed, coddle in, and enjoy happy dreams. Naturally, this depends upon the place and/or activity the patient selected the day before. With children, a mask induction can be made very interesting with all sorts of relevant suggestions, such as "going up in a space ship or wearing a mask to inhale additional oxygen, while diving in the ocean to see all the interesting creatures living there."

It is advantageous to remind patients of all the important ways they have learned to help their bodies to relax muscle tissues, to lose less blood by shunting it away from the operative areas, and in general to retain proper homeostasis. Repeated reassurance of our presence and of watching all their vital signs and making sure that they are safe and comfortable goes a long way. This method is known as " talking the patient to sleep."

During Surgery

The same hypnotic techniques can be used whenever it is necessary to communicate with patients during anesthetic unconsciousness. Calling patients by their first name, and in a very low voice reassuring them that all is well and making appropriate suggestions will be perceived by them. There is ample evidence that anesthetized patients not only hear or perceive what is being said, but they carry the effects of these perceptions along with them after surgery in the presence of dense amnesia (Cheek, 1964; Levinson, 1965; Pearson, 1961; Wolfe & Millet, 1960; Cheek's review of the literature 1959–79: Awareness of Meaningful Sounds under General Anesthesia: Considerations and a Review of the Literature, in H.J. Wain, 1981, p. 87; Rogers & Reich, 1986; Bennet, 1988) to name just a few. Changes in blood pressure and/or heart rate, for which there is no other reason, can be detected easily. In such a case, it is necessary to communicate with the patient with reassuring words, and invariably these changes reverse without any other intervention. It is remarkable to see how patients can respond to commands given by physicians with whom they are familiar and whom they trust, even though they are adequately anesthetized. Even when there is no pressing need to communicate with patients during surgery, it is advisable to maintain contact with them in such a way. When patients are losing too much blood from oozing during major surgery, one may tell them that their body knows how to stop bleeding, that they have done it many times previously and they need to do it right now. This reminds patients of previous injuries or nosebleeds and how they possibly helped their body to stop the bleeding while relaxing and letting the normal physiological reactions proceed. In cases like this, David Cheek, would lean over the screen and address his patients by their first name commanding them to "stop this nonsense and send your blood to other parts of your body," and they did (personal communication). Clawson (1975, p 162) did the same thing with his grandson. When the latter bled extensively, he commanded him to stop that bleeding and the boy promptly did.

The aim is to protect patients, keep them psychologically and physiologically stable by reinforcing suggestions made previously, using hypnotic techniques during the entire surgical period.

During Emergence from Anesthesia

During completion of surgery, a prompt emergence from anesthesia is assured by talking to patients, telling them that surgery is almost completed, that they did very well and that in a few minutes it will be time for them to wake up promptly and comfortably, pleased and surprised how quickly the time had passed. As anesthesia lightens, such suggestions are accepted invariably, because patients are still very suggestible at that time. Depending upon the situation, it is important to inform patients of the presence and purpose of various apparatus, such as an endotracheal tube, a respirator, catheters, intravenous administration of blood, etc. Patients need to understand the purpose and action of these devices and that all this was planned and not instituted because of some mishap. They might have forgotten that they were prepared for this during the preoperative visit and such explanations will reassure them. It is very frightening for a patient to wake up and not to be able to talk because the endotracheal tube is still in place, or the patient might feel pain in their bladder due to the presence of a urinary catheter.

There are some situations which need special considerations. For example, with cancer surgery, the patient has to be protected from careless remarks and from words that the patient might misinterpret. This can be accomplished by programming the patient to pay attention to the anesthesiologist's or surgeon's voice and only when addressed by name. Everything else will be background noise, such as the results of frozen sections, which often are transmitted to the surgical suite over the intercom system. Obviously, patients need to be informed about the results, but this should be done in the kindest way possible. For instance, at the end of surgery, when the patient is still groggy from the anesthetic, the patient might be told that the tumor has been removed and from now on the immune system can take care of any remaining cells, should there be any. Patients can also be reminded that they can play a very important role in helping their body to strengthen their immune system and heal rapidly. Children react well to very graphic explanations and to stories about the white knights who are fighting the black knights and how they are gobbling them up. Such explanations need to be appropriate and interesting to them.

It is not surprising that several years ago, when anethesiologists first started to talk to patients during surgery, surgeons were either dubious or were worried that "their patients," were not properly anesthetized. However, when, after a relatively short time, they observed that "their patients" did remarkably well, their attitude changed and they respected them, not only for caring so much for "their patients," but also for the extra time they thought was needed to accomplish such improvements. It has been shown that it takes no additional time to teach these very willing patients who are in a state of increased suggestibility. It also is very gratifying to see empirically-used hypnotic techniques and suggestions validated by research, and by well-controlled clinical studies which appeared during the last 30 or 40 years (Barber, 1977; Evans & Richardson, 1988; Kleinhouse & Solomon, 1995; Lynn, 1997).

Previously, anesthesiologists had the luxury of routinely seeing their patients the night before surgery. Today, in most hospitals, even major surgical procedures are done in an outpatient facility and patients are admitted the day of surgery. However, in most instances, it is possible to arrange a 10- to 15-minute interview with patients, which usually is enough time to prepare them with the use of hypnotic techniques. The reward for this is well worth the effort.

On the Way to the Recovery Room

While wheeling the patients to the recovery room, the anesthesiologist should continuously talk to them, reminding them of all the things they have told them before. This is an excellent way to use the time of emergence from chemical anesthesia for repeating positive, constructive suggestions. By now, patients may already realize that a number of things have come true, such as having awakened comfortably from anesthesia and being surprised that surgery took so little time. It is wonderful to see how amicable and grateful these patients are. There is excellent rapport between the patient and the physician and the likelihood of legal action, even in case of maloccurance, appears diminished. It seems that only patients who are angry and feel neglected are inclined to sue.

In the Recovery Room

It is reassuring to tell patients that the surgery has been completed, healing has begun, that they can be very comfortable, and that they will feel thirsty and hungry in a very short time. The nurses are instructed not to put an emesis basin on the patient's bed. This would imply that the patient will experience nausea or even vomiting. The repetition of suggestions made previously, that all bodily functions will return promptly, that it will be easy to gain control of their bladder and bowel, and that they can look forward to a speedy and complete recovery, is very valuable. Frequently, patients also notice with pleasure that they can be much more comfortable than they anticipated. Not only will they enjoy all the good care they will receive, but they will also be able to return to their home sooner than they anticipated. Most patients will have an intravenous catheter in place, and an explanation that the fluid or the blood which they are receiving is also speeding their recovery will be comforting to them. If an endotracheal tube is in place, they should be reminded of its purpose even though it was explained during the preoperative visit. The same holds true of the respirator or any other tubes or apparatus. This is of great importance, especially when patients find themselves, or one of their extremities in an uncomfortable or unusual position, such as we see sometimes in orthopedic surgery. If they feel certain sensations in the operative area, this will be a sign that healing has begun and they should relax this area so there is no pull on the sutures, which will make them more comfortable. Last but not least, they are encouraged to go to their favorite place or any other relaxing and enjoyable location frequently, that this will not only contribute to their comfort, but it also will promote healing and shorten their hospital stay. Bensen (1971) reported excellent results using positive suggestions to his surgical patients while in the recovery room.

For the relief of pain, hypnosis and hypnotic techniques are very useful. The sensation of pain has two distinct components: (1) The organic part: the impact of the surgeon's knife, the dentist touching a nerve when working on a tooth, etc. and (2) the psychogenic part: the stress, fear, and anxiety, which may be present to varying degrees. Pain is an interplay between the patient's biological, psychological, and cultural make-up. The perception of pain depends upon the personal experience, the emotional and psychological state at the moment, the memory of past pain experiences, expectation for relief, the general outlook, the perception of control (Pennebaker, Burnam, Scharffer & Harper, 1977), and the severity of stress (Chapman & Turner, 1986). In hypnosis, we process images, which allows us to modulate perception (Spiegel, 1997). In the perception of pain, it is not only the actual physical impact but, most importantly, the psychological meaning and the reaction to it. It is more important to assess the quality and the psychodynamic background of the pain, rather than its severity. Beecher (1956) has shown so decisively the difference in the requirements of narcotics following injuries in civilian life, as compared to identical injuries in the battlefield. Only one-third of the soldiers required narcotics, compared to all civilians who requested them. The soldiers had a positive outlook; they knew they would be taken care of and possibly even sent home. The meaning, the reaction, and the interpretation of the injured have a great influence upon their perception of pain. It is the stress, which hurts more, rather than the nociceptive part of the sensation. The stress, fear, and anxiety can be relieved with hypnosis, making appropriate suggestions. However, Hilgard, Morgan & McDonald (1975a) have shown experimentally that there is always a part of the person (possibly the ego) that is unconsciously aware of what is going on. He named it "the hidden observer." There is a physiological response to pain, such as an increase in heart rate and blood pressure, during cold pressor tests. In hypnotic analgesia, there is an incongruence between verbal reports and involuntary measures. This is a very interesting finding, since the subjects do not report pain on a conscious level and they are not aware of any change in vital signs. Wickramasekera (1997, p. 277) concludes that pain perception is not abolished but only attenuated. One could wonder if he had used ideomotor finger signals, whether there would have been a positive response. It is wise to remember the "hidden observer" postoperatively, when hypertension and/or an increase in heart rate occurs, which has no obvious cause. A small dose of a narcotic will correct the situation promptly.

With surgical patients, if there is pain, it is acute and can be treated promptly and easily following surgery. However, at times, chronic pain may present a problem if the pain is still present after corrective surgery, such as after laminectomy for chronic back pain. Under these circumstances, the whole personality of the patient must be evaluated to determine the amount of secondary gain the pain represents to this patient. If there is litigation involved in case of an accident or malpractice, the patient may subconsciously not be willing to give up the pain after surgery.

Hypnotically-prepared patients need minimal narcotics postoperatively. When using self-hypnosis, they are able to go to their favorite place any time they feel the slightest discomfort. Nurses in the recovery room are instructed never to ask patients whether they have pain. Patients should be told that they may ask for medications in case they should be uncomfortable and not able to regain comfort on their own. As mentioned previously, the word "pain" should never be used, because it may remind patients of traumatic experiences involving severe pain, which they may have encountered in the past.

Hypnotic techniques can also be used when minor surgical procedures, or painful invasive maneuvers need to be performed. They help with examinations which might be painful and require relaxation and the cooperation of the patient, such as endoscopies and vaginal or rectal examinations. Patients can be made comfortable with specific hypnotic suggestions and these procedures can be performed with greater ease and safety when the patient is in a hypnotic state. Lang, Joyce, and Spiegel (1996) describe beautifully very similar results with patients inducing "self-hypnotic relaxation."

Results

When patients are prepared with hypnosis and when these techniques are used during induction, during surgery, and in the recovery room, anxiety and stress are reduced considerably. Following chemical anesthesia, these patients wake up comfortably and require very little or no sedation at all. Emergence delirium is not seen when patients were prepared properly with hypnotic techniques. Nausea or vomiting is rare because they feel thirsty and hungry, a suggestion which is routinely given during the preoperative visit. Williams, Hind, Sweeney, and Fisher (1994) also showed a decrease in nausea and vomiting with the use of hypnosis preoperatively. Faymonville, Fissette, Mambourg, Roedigger, Joris, and Lamy (1995), using hypnosis routinely to provide conscious sedation for plastic surgery, reported a very low incidence of nausea and vomiting postoperatively. Patients urinate promptly when their bladders are full and bowel movements will appear promptly, because normal peristalsis sets in soon after completion of the surgery. Even after hemorrhoidectomies, the elimination is less painful, because patients were taught to relax their rectal sphincter, so stool can pass easily. Disbrow, Bennett, and Owings (1993) showed that patients who received specific suggestions preoperatively, as a result had significantly shorter return of intestinal motility than patients who were given nonspecific suggestions.

In general, patients have a much smoother postoperative course, fewer pulmonary complications, and less frequent infections. They also leave the hospital an average of two days earlier than patients who just experienced a routine preoperative visit without the use of hypnotic techniques (Evans & Richardson, 1988). Hart (1980) reported that patients listening to a tape with hypnotic suggestions preoperatively and undergoing cardiac surgery showed lower diastolic pressures, needed fewer transfusions, and were much calmer postoperatively than patients in the control group. This is even more remarkable because most practitioners believe that patients who are prepared with a commercial tape do not do as well as patients who experience hetero-hypnosis prior to surgery. Patients with advanced breast cancer showed remarkable results when hypnosis was used (Spiegel, Kraemer, Bloom, and Gottheil, 1989). Their quality of life improved perceptibly as well as their survival rate. Blankfield (1991) reviewed the literature dealing with "Suggestion, Relaxation, and Hypnosis as Adjuncts in the Care of Surgery Patients" and showed significant differences in a variety of parameters such as nausea and vomiting, prompt return of physiological functions, decrease in the use of narcotics, decrease of infections, hospital stay, etc. Only two out of seventeen papers reported no significant difference between treatment groups and control groups, namely Surman, Hacket, Silverberg, and Behrendt (1974) and Abramson, Greenfield, and Heron (1968). Also Liu, Standen, and Aitkenhead (1992) also reported no difference in postoperative outcome nor in length of hospital stay. In most of these studies, commercial tapes were used for the induction and for giving various suggestions. It is so much more powerful when a human being, who has established rapport with the patient, induces hypnosis and makes appropriate suggestions. Patients are very sensitive and perceive the personal involvement of the physician. Cohen and Lazarus (1973) and Kornfield, Heller, Frank, and Moskowitz (1974) observed that avoidant patients who are not concerned about details preoperatively do better than vigilant patients who want to control and be informed about everything.

The routine use of hypnotic techniques has a great influence, not only on the emotional well-being of patients but also on physical parameters. It is known that psychological problems can produce psychosomatic symptoms and even diseases. It is also believed that psychological procedures can lead to psychosomatic well-being. With the elimination of stress, anxiety, and fear, the natural capacity of the body to heal is not impaired and with appropriate therapeutic suggestions psycho-physiological healing and well-being is promoted. Besides this, the savings in the cost of hospitalization can be considerable. This has gained a great deal of significance in today's health care system, where costs per patient seem to be of overriding importance.

Unfortunately, psychological preparation as described in the previous pages is practiced only in rare instances and as a rule only upon the request of a patient, a surgeon, or a very knowledgeable and trained anesthesiologist. The psychological, physiological, and monitary advantages of hypnosis preoperatively, during surgery, and postoperatively have been used and documented for at least 30 years (Kessler & Dane, 1996). As early as 1894, Cocke wrote, "I earnestly hope that a widespread effort on the part of the surgeons, both in Europe and America, will bring about a more intelligent application of it (hypnosis) and ameliorate much suffering which now goes unrelieved." Unfortunately, this has not happened. Fellows (1996) made a survey of the teaching of hypnosis in British psychology departments and found the situation deplorable even though the "attitudes towards teaching and research in hypnosis remained very positive, and over 80% of returns indicated a perception of hypnosis as a suitable topic for research and teaching." The situation in the United States is no different, although there seems to be some progress as far as the frequency of seminars and workshops is concerned. In 1959, hypnosis became mainstream medicine in the United States with the report of the AMA Council on Mental Health recognition of it as a legitimate medical modality. Many people erroniously perceived it as "alternative" medicine.

Hypnotic techniques should be an integral part of the practice of surgery and anesthesiology, as well as of all other medical specialties. It is regrettable that we have not been able to teach this valuable technique to our medical students, interns, and most residents, in order to give patients the advantages we have observed for so many years. We should include the teaching of medical hypnosis in the curriculum of medical schools, internships, and residency programs. If this could be implemented, we would be able not only to help our patients, but also to reduce the cost of medical care. The hope is that with the publication of this book and with the interest it should arouse, the use of medical hypnosis will become widespread.

REFERENCES

Abramson, M., Greenfield, L., & Heron, W.T. (1968). Response to or perception of auditory stimuli under deep surgical anesthesia. *American Journal of Obstetrics and Gynecology, 96:* 584–585.

Auerbach, S.M. (1989). Stress management and coping research in the health care setting: An overview and methological commentary. *Journal of Consulting Clinical Psychology, 57* (3): 388–395.

Bakan, P. (1969). Hypnotizability, laterality of eye movement and functioal brain asymmetry. Perceptual and motor skills, 28, 927–932. In K.S. Bowers (1983), *Hypnosis for the seriously curious.* New York-London: W.W. Norton.

Barber J. (1993): The clinical role of responsivity tests: A master class commentary. *American Journal of Clinical and Experimental Hypnosis, 41*(3), p. 165.

Barber, J. (1996). *Hypnosis and suggestion in the treatment of pain.* London: W. W. Norton & Co.

Barber, J. (1977). Rapid induction analgesia: A clinical report. *American Journal of Clinical Hypnosis, 19:* 138–147.

Bartlett, E.E. (1966). Polypharmacy versus hypnosis in surgical patients. *Pacific Medicine and Surgery, 74,* 109–112.

Bartlett, E.E. (1971). The use of hypnotic techniques without hypnosis per se for temporary stress. *American Journal of Clinical Hypnosis, 13:* 273–278.

Beecher, H.K. (1956). Relationship of significance of wound to pain experienced. *Journal of the American Medical Association, 161:* 1609–1613.

Bennett H.L. (1988). Perception and memory for events during adequate general anesthesia for surgical operation. In H.M. Pettinati (Ed.) *Hypnosis and memory.* New York: Guilford, pp. 193–231.

Bennett, H.L., Benson, D.R., & Kuiken, D.A. (1986). Preoperative instructions for decreased bleeding during spine surgery. *Anesthesiology, 65*(3A), A245.

Bennett, H.L., Davis, H.S., & Giannini, J.A. (1985). Non-verbal response to intraoperative conversation. *British Journal of Anesthesia, 57*(2), 174–179.

Bensen, V.B. (1971). One hundred cases of post-anesthetic suggestion in the recovery room. *American Journal of Clinical Hypnosis, 14*(1) 9–15.

Bishay, E.G., (1984). Studies of the effects of hypnoanesthesia on regional blood flow by transcutaneous oxygen monitoring. *American Journal of Clinical Hypnosis, 27*(1), 64–69.

Black, P.H., (1994). Immune system-central nervous system interactions: Psychoneuroendocrinology of stress and its immune consequences. *Antimicrobial*

Agents and Chemotherapy, 38, 1–6.

Blankfield, R. P. (1991). Suggestion, relaxation, and hypnosis as adjuncts in the care of surgery patients: A review of the literature. *American Journal of Clinical Hypnosis, 33*(3), 172–186.

Bonke, B., Fitsh, W., & Millar, K. (Eds.). (1990). *Memory and awareness in anesthesia.* Amsterdam: Swets & Zeitlinger.

Bonke, B., Smitz, P., Verhage, F., & Zwageling, A. (1986). Clinical study of so-called unconscious perception during general anesthesia. *British Journal of Anesthesia, 58*(9), 957–964.

Breckenridge, J.L., & Aitkenhead, A.R. (1983). Awareness during anesthesia: A review. *Annals Royal College of Surgery,* 65, 93–101.

Brunn, J.T. (1963). The capacity to hear, understand and to remember personal experiences during chemo-anesthesia: A personal experience. *American Journal of Clinical Hypnosis,* 6, 27–30.

Casiglia, E., Mazza, A., Ginnocchio, G., Onesto C., Pessina, A.C., Rossi, A., Cavatton, G., & Marotti, A. (1997). Hemodynamics in real and hypnosis-simulated phlebotomy. *American Journal of Clinical Hypnosis, 40*(1) 368–375.

Chapman, C.R., & Turner, J.A. (1986). Psychological control of acute pain in medical settings. *Journal of Pain Symptom Management, 1,* 9–20.

Chaves, J.F. (1980). Hypnotic control of surgical bleeding. Paper presented at the Annual Meeting of the American Psychological Association, Montreal, Quebec, Canada, September 1980.

Cheek, D.B. (1965). Can surgical patients react to what they hear under anesthesia? *Journal of the American Assocciation of House Anesthesiologists,* February 1965, 36–38.

Cheek, D.B. (1959). Subconscious perception of meaningful sounds during surgical anesthesia as reviewed under hypnosis. *American Journal of Clinical Hypnosis, 1*(3), 102–113.

Cheek, D.B. (1960). Use of preoperative hypnosis to protect patients from careless conversation. *American Journal of Clinical Hypnosis, 3*(2), 101–102.

Cheek, D.B. (1962b). Some applications of hypnosis and ideomotor questioning methods for analysis and therapy in medicine. *American Journal of Clinical Hypnosis, 5*(2), 92.

Cheek, D.B. (1964). Further evidence of persistence of hearing under chemo-anesthesia: Detailed case report. *American Journal of Clinical Hypnosis, 7*(1), 55–59.

Cheek, D.B. (1962a). The importance of recognizing that surgical patients behave as though hypnotized. *American Journal of Clinical Hypnosis, 4*(4), 227.

Clawson, T.A., Jr., & Swade, R.H. (1975). The hypnotic control of blood flow and pain: The cure of warts and the potential for the use of hypnosis in the treatment of cancer. *American Journal of Clinical Hypnosis, 17*(3),160–164.

Cocke, J.R., (1894). *Hypnotism.* Boston: Arena.

Coe, W.C., Peterson, P., & Gwynn, M. (1995). Expectations and sequelae to hypnosis: Initial findings. *American Journal of Clinical Hypnosis, 38*(1) 3–12.

Cohen, F., & Lazarus, R.S. (1973). Active coping processes, coping dispositions, and recovery from surgery. *Psychosomatic Medicine,* 35, 375–389.

Dillon, M., Minchoff, B. & Baker, K. H. (1985). Positive emotional states and enhancement of the immune system. *International Journal of Psychiatry in Medicine, 15:*1, 13–18.

Disbrow, E.A., Bennet, H.L., & Owings, J.T. (1993): Effect of preoperative suggestion on postoperative motility. *Western Journal of Medicine, 158*(5), 488–492.

Dubin, L.L., & Shapiro, S.S. (1977). Use of hypnosis to faciliate dental extraction in a classic hemophiliac with a high antibody titer to factor VIII. *American Journal of Clinical Hypnosis, 20*(1), 79–83.

Duke, J. (1968). Lateral eye-movement behavior. *Journal of General Psychology, 78,* 189–195.

Dumas, R.G., & Leonard, R.C. (1963). The effect of nursing on the incidence of postoperative vomiting. *Nursing Res, 12,* 15.

Egbert, L. D., Battit, G.E., & Turndorf, H. (1963): The value of the preoperative visit by the anesthetist: A study of doctor patient rapport. *Journal of the American Medical Association, 185,* 553–555.

Egbert, L. D., Battit, G. E., Welch, C. E., & Bartlett, E. E. (1964). Reduction of postoperative pain by encouragement and instruction of patients. *New England Journal of Medicine, 270*(16): 825–827.

Enqvist, B., & Ficher, (1997). Preoperative hypnotic techniques reduce consumption of analgesics after surgical removal of third mandibular molars. *The International Journal of Clinical and Experimental Hypnosis, 45*(2), 102–108.

Enqvist, B., Konow, L., & Bystedt, H. (1995). Pre- and perioperative suggestion in maxillofacial surgery. Effects on blood loss and recovery. *The International Journal of Clinical and Experimental Hypnosis, 43*(3), 284–293.

Enqvist, B., Konow, L., & Bystedt, H. (1996). Stress reduction, preoperative hypnosis and perioperative suggestion in mxillo-facial surgery: Somatic responses and recovery. *Hypnos, 23*(2), 76–82.

Erickson, M., (1982). Ericksonian approaches to hypnosis and psychotherapy. In Zweig, J. (Ed.), AV/QY: New York : Brunner-Mazel.

Erickson, M.H., (1980). Literalness: An experimental study. In E. Rossi (Ed.). *The collected papers of Milton H. Erickson on hypnosis* (Vol.3) Hypnotic investigation of psychodynamic processes. New York: Irvington.

Erickson, M.H., (1965). An introduction to the study and application of hypnosis for pain control. Presented at the International Congress of Hypnosis and Psychosomatic Medicine. Paris, France.

Evans, B., & Stanley R. (1991). Hypnoanesthesia and hypnotic techniques with surgical patients. *Australian Journal of Clinical and Experimental Hypnosis,19*(1), 31–39.

Evans, C., & Richardson, P. (1988). Improved recovery and reduced postoperative stay after therapeutic suggestions under general anesthesia. *Lancet, II:* 491–493.

Ewin, D. (1994). Many memories retrieved with hypnosis are accurate. *American Journal of Clinical Hypnosis, 36*(3), p175.

Ewin, D.M., (1984). Hypnosis in surgery and anesthesia. In W.C. Wester & A.H. Smith (Eds.), *Clinical hypnosis-A multidisciplinary approach.* Philadelphia: J.B. Lippincott, pp. 210–235.

Faymonville, M.E., Fissette, J., Mambourg, P.H., Roediger, L., Joris, J., & Lamy, M. (1995). Hypnosis as adjunct therapy in conscious sedation for plastic sugery.

Regional Anesthesia, 20(2), 145.

Fellows, B.J. (1996). Teaching hypnosis in British psychology departments: A 10-year follow-up. *Contemporary Hypnosis, 13*(2), 74–79.

Field, P. (1974). Effects of tape-recorded hypnotic preparation for surgery. *International Journal of Clinical and Experimental Hypnosis, 22:* 54–61.

Fortin, F., & Kirouac, S. (1976). A randomized controlled trial of preoperative patient education. *International Journal Nursing Studies 13*, 11–24.

Fredericks, L.E. (1967). The use of hypnosis in hemophilia. *American Journal of Clinical Hypnosis, 10*(1), 52–55.

Fredericks, L.E. (1980). The value of teaching hypnosis in the practice of anesthesiology. *The International Journal of Clinical and Experimental Hypnosis, 28*(1), 6–14.

Fredericks, L.E. (1988). Hypnoanesthesia and preparation for surgery. American Society for Clinical Hypnosis, 30th Annual Scientific Meeting and Workshop in Clinical Hypnosis, Chicago, IL, USA.

Fredericks, L.E. (1978). Teaching of hypnosis in the overall approach to the surgical patient. *American Journal of Clinical Hypnosis, 20*(3), 175–183.

Goldman, L., Ogg, T.W., & Levey, A.B. (1988). Hypnosis and daycare anesthesia: A study to reduce pre-operative anxiety and intra-operative anesthetic requirements. *Anesthesia, 43*, 466–469.

Grabowska, M.J. (1971). The effect of hypnosis and hypnotic suggestions on the blood flow in the extremities. *Polish Medical Journal, 10*, 044–1051.

Greenleaf, M., Fisher, S., Miaskowski, C., & DuHamel, K. (1992). Hypnotisability and recovery from cardiac surgery. *American Journal of Clinical Hypnosis, 35*(2), 119–128.

Hart, R.R., (1980). The influence of a taped hypnotic induction treatment procedure on the recovery of surgery patients. *International Journal of Clinical and Experimental Hypnosis, 28*(4), 324–332.

Hilgard, E.R., & Hilgard, J.R. (1983). *Hypnosis in the relief of pain.* Los Altos, CA: William Kaufman, pp. 120–143.

Hilgard, E.R., Morgan, A.H., & McDonald, H. (1975a). Pain and dissociation in the cold pressor test: A study of hypnotic analgesia with "hidden reports" through automatic key-pressing and automatic talking. *Journal of Abnormal Psychology, 84*, 280–289.

Houge, D.R. (1997). A model for the application of hypnotic techniques for anesthesia during surgery. Clinical hypnosis as the sole form of anesthesia in orthopedic surgery. The 14th International Congress of Hypnosis, San Diego, CA.

Houghton, L.A., Heyman, D.J., & Whorwell, P.J. (1996). Symptomatology, quality of life and economic features of irritable bowel syndrome: The effect of hypnotherapy. *Alimentary Pharmacology & Therapeutics, 10*(1), 91–95.

Howard, J.F. (1987). Incidents of auditory perception during anesthesia with traumatic sequelae. *Medical Journal Australia, 146*(1), 44–46.

Johnson, V.C., Walker, L.G., Heys, S.D., Whiting, P.H., & Eremin, O. (1996). Can relaxation training and hypnotherapy modify the immune response to stress, and is hypnotizability relevant? *Contemporary Hypnosis, 13*(2), 100–108.

Johnston, M. (1980). Anxiety in surgical patients. *Psychological Medicine, 10*, 145–152.

Jones, J., & Konieczko, K. (1986). Hearing and memory in anesthetized patients. *British Medical Journal, 292*, 1291–1293.

Kessler, R., & Dane J.R. (1996). Psychological and hypnotic preparation for anesthesia and surgery. *International Journal of Clinical and Experimental Hypnosis, 44*(3), 189–207.

Kessler, R. (1997). The consequences of individual differences in preparation for surgery and invasive medical procedures. *Hypnosis, XXIV*, 4, 181–192.

Kihlstrom, J.F., Evans, F.G., Orne, E.C., & Orne, M.T. (1980). Attempting to breach post hypnotic amnesia. *Journal of Abnormal Psychology, 89*(5) 603–616.

Kihlstrom, J.F., & Schachter, D.L. (1990). Anesthesia, amnesia and the cognitive unconscious. In B. Bonke, W. Fitch, & K. Millar (Eds.), *Memory and awareness in anaesthesia.* Amsterdam: Swets & Zeitlinger, pp 21–44.

Kirsch, I. (1994). Clinical hypnosis as a non deceptive placebo: Empirically derived techniques. *American Journal of Clinical Hypnosis, 37*(2), 95–106.

Klein, K.B., & Spiegel, D. (1989). Modulation of gastric acid secretion by hypnosis. *Gastroenterology, 96*, 1383–1387.

Kleinhauz, M., & Solomon, Z. (1995). Hypnotherapeutic approaches and outcome of combat stress reactions 18 years later. Part 1: Clinical description and treatment strategies. *Hypnosis International Monographs, 1*, 145–152.

Kolough, F.T. (1968). The frightened surgical patient. *American Journal of Clinical Hypnosis, 11*(20), 89.

Kornfield, D.S., Heller, S.S., Frank, K.A., & Moskowitz, R. (1974). Personality and psychological factors in postcardiotomy delirium. *Archives of General Psychiatry, 31*, 249–253.

LaBaw, W.L., (1975). Auto-Hypnosis in haemophilia. *Haematologie: International Quaterly of Haematologia, 9*(1–2), 103–110.

Lang, E.V., Joyce, J.S., Spiegel, D., Hamilton, D., & Lee, K.K. (1996). Self-hypnotic relaxation during interventional radiological procedures: Effects on pain perception and intravenous drug use. *The International Journal of Clinical and Experimental Hypnosis, Vol. 44*(2), 106–119.

Lazarus, H.R., & Hagens, J.H. (1968). Prevention of psychosis following open heart surgery. *American Journal of Psychiatry, 124*, 1190–1195.

Levinson, B.W. (1965). States of awareness under general anesthesia. *British Journal of Anaesthesiology, 37*, 544–546.

Liu, W.H., Standen, P.J., & Aitkenhead, A.R. (1992): Therapeutic suggestions during general anesthesia in patients undergoing hyterectomy. *British Journal of Anaesthesiology, 68*(3), 277–281.

Lucas, O.N., (1965). Dental extractions in the hemophiliac, control of emotional factors by hypnosis. *American Journal of Clinical Hypnosis, 7*, 301–307.

Lynn, S.J. (1997). Hypnosis and memory: A workshop. 14th International Congress of Hypnosis. San Diego, CA.

Magaw, A. (1906). A review of over fourteen thousand surgical anesthetics. *Surgery, Gynecology & Obstetrics, 3*:795–797.

Mark, J.B., & Greenberg, L.M. (1983). Intraoperative awareness and hypertensive crisis during high-dose Fentanyl-Oxigen anesthesia. *Anesthesia and Analgesia, 62*, 698.

McLintock, T.T.C., Aitken, H., Downie, C.F.A., & Kenney, G.N.C. (1990). Postoperative analgesic requirements in patients exposed to positive intraoperative suggestions. *British Medical Journal, 301,* 788–790.

Miller, N.E. (1969). Learning of visceral and glandular responses. *Science, 163,* 434–445.

Mishkin, M., & Petri, H. (1984). Memories and habits: Some implications for the analysis of learning and retention. In S. Squire & N. Butters (Eds.), *Neuropsychology of memory.* New York: Guilford, pp. 287–296.

Mittleman, K.D., Doubt, T.J., & Gravitz, M.A. (1992). Influence of self-induced hypnosis on thermal responses during emersion in 25 degrees C water. *Aviation Space & Environmental Medicine, 63,* 689–695.

Moore, L.E., & Wiesner, S.L. (1996). Hypnotically-induced vasodilatation in the treatment of repetitive strain injuries. *American Journal of Clinical Hypnosis, 39(2),* 97–104.

Munglani, R., & Jones, J.G. (1994): Information processing during sleep and anesthesia. *Anaesthesia Review, 10,* 107–130.

Olness, K. (1997). Symposium: Pediatric uses of hypnosis: Mastcell activation in juvenile migraineurs who learn self-hypnosis. The 14th International Congress of Hypnosis, San Diego, CA.

Olness, K., Culbert, T., & Uden, D. (1989). Self-regulation of salivary immunoglobulin A by children. *Pediatrics, 83,* 66–71.

Pearson R.E. (1961). Response to suggestions given during general anesthesia. *American Journal of Clinical Hypnosis, 4*(2), 106–114.

Pearson, R.E. (1973). Lecture given at the Institute of the Pennsylvania Hospital, Philadelphia, PA., February 1973.

Pennebaker, J.W., Burnam, M.A., Schaeffer, M.A., & Harper, D.C. (1977). Lack of control as a determinant of perceived physical symptoms. *Journal of Personal Social Psychology, 35,* 167–174.

Pert, C. (1997). Molecules of emotion. *Why you feel the way you feel.* New York: Scribner.

Peter, B. (1998). Normal instruction or hypnotic suggestion: What makes the difference? *Hypnosis, 25:* 61–71.

Quirk, M.E., Letendre, A.J., Ciottone, R.A., & Ligley, J.F. (1989). Anxiety of patients undergoing MRI imaging. *Radiology, 170,* 463–466.

Ridgeway, V., & Mathews, A. (1982). Psychological preparation for surgery. A comparison of methods. *British Journal of Clinical Psychology, 21,* 271–280.

Rodger, B.P. (1961). The art of preparing the patient for anesthesia. *Anesthesiology, 22*(4), 548–554.

Rogers M., & Reich P. (1986). Psychological intervention with surgical patients: Evaluation and outcome. *Advanced Psychosomatic Medicine, 15,* 23–50.

Rossi, E.L., & Cheek, D.B. (1990). Summary steps for preoperative hypnosis to facilitate healing. In D. Hammond (Ed.), *Handbook of hypnotic suggestions and metaphors.* New York: W.W. Norton.

Rossi, E.L., & Cheek, D.B. (1988). *Mind-body therapy: Ideodynamic healing in hypnosis.* New York: W.W. Norton.

Salmon, P. (1992). Surgery as a psychological stressor: Paradoxical effects of preoperative emotional state and endocrine resposes. *Stress Medicine, 8,* 193–198.

Sime, A.M. (1976). Relationship of preoperative fear, type of coping, and information received about surgery to recover from surgery. *Journal Personal Social Psychology, 34*(4), 716–724.

Smith, P., Barabasz, A., Barabasz, M., & Warner, D. (1995). Effects of hypnosis on the immune response: B-cells, T-cells, helper and suppressor cells. *American Journal Clinical Hypnosis, 38*:2, 71–79.

Spiegel, D. (1997). Hypnosis: Physiology, psychology and performance. The 14th International Congress of Hypnosis, San Diego, CA.

Spiegel, D., Kraemer, H.C., Bloom, L.R., & Gottheil, E. (1989). Effect of psychological survival of patients with metastatic breast cancer. *Lancet, 2,* 8668, 888–891.

Spielberger, C.D. (1973). Emotional reactions to surgery. *Journal of Consulting Clinical Psychologists, 40*(1), 33.

Surman, O.S., Hacket, T.P., Silverberg, E.L., & Behrendt, D.M. (1974). Usefulness of psychiatric intervention in patients undergoing cardiac surgery. *Archives of General Psychiatry, 30,* 830–835.

Swersky-Saechetti, T., & Margolis, C.J. (1986). The effects of a comprehensive self-hypnosis training program in the use of factor VIII in severe hemophilia. *International Journal of Clinical and Experimental Hypnosis, 34*(2), 71–83.

Torem, M.S. (1992). "Back from the future": A powerful age-progression technique. *American Journal of Clinical Hypnosis, 35*(2), 81–98.

Wain, J. J. (1981). Theoretical and clinical aspects of hypnosis. Miami, Florida. *Symposia Specialists.*

Weinberger, N.M., Gold, P.E., & Sternberg, D.B. (1984). Epinephrine enables Pavlovian fear conditioning under anesthesia. *Science, 223,* 605–607.

Wickramasekera, I. (1997). Editorial commentary on hypnotic suggestion: A musical metaphor. *American Journal of Clinical Hypnosis, 39*(4), p 277.

Williams, A.R. Hind, M. Sweeney, B.P., & Fisher, R. (1994). Incidence and severity of postoperative nausea and vomiting in patients exposed to positive intraoperative suggestions. *Anaesthesia, 49*(4), 340–342.

Wolfe L., & Millet J. (1960). Control of postoperative pain by suggestion under general anesthesia. *American Journal of Clinical Hypnosis 3*(2), 109–112.

Yapko, M.D. (1990). Trancework. New York: Brunner/Mazel. In B.J. Walsh, (1997) Goldfinger: A framework for resolving affect using ideomotor questioning. *American Journal of Clinical Hypnosis, 40*(1), 349–359.

Yapko, M.D. (1996). An interview with David Cheek, M.D. *American Journal of Clinical Hypnosis, 39*(1), p 14.

Zimmerman, J. (1998). Hypnotic technique for sedation of patients during upper gastrointestinal endoscopy. *American Journal of Clinical Hypnosis, 40*(4), p 282.

Chapter 4

HYPNOSIS IN CONJUNCTION WITH REGIONAL ANESTHESIA

LILLIAN E. FREDERICKS

When patients are scheduled for surgery and regional anesthesia is the method of choice, they are either admitted to an outpatient facility, a short procedure unit of a hospital, or the surgery may be performed in the office of a surgeon. The pressure and immediacy which are prevalent in the emergency situation or when patients are admitted to a hospital for major surgery are not present because these procedures are planned and scheduled. As a rule, the amount of anxiety, stress, and apprehension is considerably less than in patients who have to undergo surgery with chemical anesthesia involving the loss of consciousness. However, there is still the threat of a diagnosis of malignancy, or the expectation of pain during or after the procedure as well as the uncertainty of the final result and outcome of the surgery.

Many hundreds of minor and major surgical procedures have been performed in the past, using hypnosis as the sole anesthetic (Esdaile, 1846–1957; Gauld, 1988). Today most minor surgical procedures are performed with regional or local anesthesia and are complemented by the use of intravenous anesthesia or sedation combined with narcotics. Because of convenience and ease of administration, most surgeons use this technique almost routinely. In today's jargon, this is called MAC (Monitored Anesthesia Care). This is relatively inexpensive, easy to administer, and does not require the surgeon to have the knowledge and expertise of using hypnosis, nor does it require the presence of another person, skilled in this modality. A nurse can be present and occasionally check the patient's blood pressure while circulating and performing other duties. One of the disadvantages in using intravenous medications is a possible drop in blood pressure, cardiovascular instability, drowsiness and respiratory depression leading to oxygen desaturation, nausea and vomiting. Because the amount of drugs given to a patient is rather arbitrary and often does not correspond to the level of stress and anxiety of each particular patient, nor to the extent of the surgery, patients may receive excessive amounts of medication and show serious side effects of these drugs, most frequently as soon as the stimulation of the surgery stops.

There are no side effects with the use of hypnosis or any other non-pharmacological sedation such as acupuncture. Tinterow (1960) wrote that hypnosis is the only means of anesthesia which carries no danger to the patient. Schultz-Stubner (1996) uses hypnosis instead of cerebral sedatives, especially for high-risk patients, because hypnosis has no side effects. In hypnosis, patients enjoy the experience of altered awareness, and with time distortion, they can undergo many hours of extensive surgery without being aware of the length of time and the discomfort of having to lie perfectly still for such a protracted period of time.

The use of hypnosis and the methods which should be used are similar to those described in previous chapters. The method of induction might differ, because patients are not as likely to be in a state of altered awareness, as is seen in emergency situations, or when patients are admitted to a hospital for major surgery. It is important to separate those patients who are in such a state, from those who are not, and act accordingly. It is advantageous to work with patients prior to the scheduled surgery, but for various reasons, this is not always possible.

Occasionally, an inadequate spinal or epidural anesthesia is encountered where the patient is suffering a good deal of pain, or the area where the surgery has to be performed is exceedingly large and the amount of local anesthetic required would be too great and possibly toxic. Under these circumstances, the use of hypnosis or hypnotic techniques is very effective. To decrease or completely eliminate the pain in the operative area is accepted by the patient willingly. At such times, the anxiety and lack of control increase the patient's suggestibility and motivation. The patient wants to feel comfortable again. The pain or discomfort is acute and the complex psychological conflicts, seen with patients with chronic pain, are absent. Since the physician and patient have not met before, it is important to quickly diagnose the problem, to be calm and collected, and establish trust and rapport with the patient. When conversing with patients, it is possible to quickly evaluate the severity of their stress and discomfort. There are many classical induction methods which can be used at this time. Most physicians have certain preferences which they use most of the time. However, the induction method, just like anything else, should be adapted to each individual patient and to the situation at hand. A rapid and frequently used technique is Spiegel's eye-roll (Spiegel & Spiegel, 1978), followed by progressive relaxation, dissociation to a specific place of comfort and preferably involving the patient into a chosen activity, which the patient then can enjoy. Following this, the patient could also be totally involved in a pleasant conversation, far apart from the situation and not paying any attention to the part of the body which needs the surgery. Eye fixation on a spot high up on a wall, or on the ceiling, raising their gaze as high as possible, which makes their eyelids tired, can also be used. This is followed by spontaneous eye closure, progressive relaxation and dissociation to a place of their choice. Other frequently used induction techniques, such as arm levitation, rigidity, or the pendulum are not appropriate for obvious reasons. The use of hypnotic techniques, without a formal induction, is often sufficient for the patient to regain control and with dissociation, with involvement of all of their senses, they can be comfortable again. The choice of words and the suggestions are crucial. One should never say, "you will be finished very soon, or it's almost over now." These phrases can easily be misinterpreted and increase their anxiety and discomfort.

It is customary practice now to admit patients on the day of surgery. These patients will have to be seen in a waiting room of the facility. There is enough time for taking a short history, establishing the coping styles of patients, an inquiry as to their likes and dislikes, and possible phobias. This should be followed by explanations of procedures which will make them safe and comfortable during the surgery. With vigilant patients, it is important to go into more details. It is not advisable to use the word "hypnosis" for reasons explained in Chapter 3. Since the patient has signed a consent for surgery and anesthesia, any technique of caring for this patient is certainly included. To talk about a very special kind of relaxation and occupying their mind with most interesting and pleasant thoughts will be readily accepted by patients. It might happen that a patient will ask "will you use hypnosis with me" or "will you hypnotize me?" In this situation, it is not appropriate to deny this, but to congratulate the patient for being so observant and one could quickly say "you probably also know how very pleasant and effective this modality is."

If at all possible, patients should be seen at least a day prior to surgery which will enable the physician or psychologist to establish rapport, teach them to enter hypnosis with a rapid induction and produce glove anesthesia, with transference of the analgesia to the operative site. This can be accomplished rather easily because it does not need a deep stage of hypnosis. Again, motivation and expectations on the part of the patient and expertise and enthusiasm on the part of the hypnotist are important.

During the surgery, it is helpful to converse with the patient in a low voice, so as not to distract or disturb the surgeon. Most patients enjoy the conversation and this kind of involvement, while others would rather sleep or just relax and pursue their own thoughts. The enthusiasm and expectancy of success on the part of everyone involved will be transmitted to the patient, and any hesitation or doubt will be perceived by the patient and interfere with the outcome. Patients are perceptive and aware of feelings, even when they are not expressed. However, these patients are very amenable to positive suggestions and accept them readily.

If during surgery, patients are experiencing pain or discomfort, it will be necessary to deepen hypnosis with appropriate deepening techniques or to use a rapid indirect induction, as described in Chapter 7. Some deepening techniques use metaphors of waves, or waterfalls, or walking down a flight of stairs and patients retreating into their special room, where they store all their sensations and turn any unwanted sensation "down, down, and down and possibly even completely off." It is necessary to use a lot of imagination, metaphors and appropriate suggestions in order to reestablish a level of comfort acceptable to the patient. When surgery has been successfully completed with the aid of hypnosis, both the patient and the surgeon are usually very pleased.

The same technique can be used to deal with patients undergoing painful invasive procedures. Lang (1996) describes a similar technique of "self-hypnotic relaxation during interventional radiological procedures" which is similar to hypnotic techniques described here.

In conclusion, it should be emphasized that in conjunction with local or regional anesthesia, there is no need to use drugs which might have undesirable side effects. Either the surgeon, an anesthesiologist, or any other healthcare practitioner trained in the use of hypnosis can make patients not only comfortable, but afford them a wonderful and rewarding experience while undergoing surgery, regardless of the extent and duration of the procedure. Today, many patients are searching for alternative approaches to pharmacological anesthesia, and the use of hypnosis can give them the added satisfaction of being able to contribute to their own well-being.

REFERENCES

Esdaile, J. (1846–1957). *Hypnosis in medicine and surgery.* (originally titled "Mesmerism in India"). New York: The Julian Press.

Gauld, A. (1988). Reflections on mesmeric analgesia. *British Journal of Experimental and Clinical Hypnosis, 5,* 17–24.

Lang, E.V., Joyce, J.S., Spiegel, D., Hamilton D., & Lee, K.K. (1996). Self-hypnotic relaxation during interventional radiological procedures: Effects on pain perception and intravenous drug use. *The International Journal of Clinical and Experimental Hypnosis, 44*(2), 106–119.

Schulz-Stubner, S. (1996). Hypnosis: A side effect-free alternative to medical sedation in regional anesthesia. *Anaesthetist, 45*(10), 956–969.

Spiegel, H., & Spiegel, D. (1978). *Trance and treatment: Clinical uses of hypnosis.* New York: Basic Books.

Tinterow, M.M. (1960). Hypnotic anesthesia for major surgical procedure. *American Surgeon, 26,* 732–737.1960.

Chapter 5

HYPNOSIS AS THE SOLE ANESTHETIC

LILLIAN E. FREDERICKS

Hypnosis was used to relieve pain during surgery long before chemical anesthesia was introduced. According to Gravitz (1988), the first documented case of surgery with hypnosis as the sole anesthetic was performed on April 12, 1829 by Jules Cloquet, a Parisian surgeon. John Elliotson, a British surgeon, performed surgery in 1843 with the use of hypnosis. At that time, it was called mesmerism, after Franz Anton Mesmer. Magnetism was very important field in physics at his time and Mesmer believed that, in humans, there was a negative magnet on one side and a positive magnet on the other side of the body. When the poles of these magnets were not in the right position to each other, illness would occur. He called this "animal magnetism" as distinguished from metal magnets. This can be considered a forerunner of hypnotism. James Esdaile (1846), a British surgeon, working in India, used hypnosis for surgery as the sole anesthetic in over 3000 cases and reported 345 major operations. According to Pulos (1980), Esdaile used the mesmeric process of inducing somatic anesthesia. It is interesting to note, as he describes that ". . . the most frequently described procedure began with the patient lying down with eyes closed. There was no preparation nor expectation, and no verbal exchange between mesmerist and patient" (p. 207). This differs greatly from present beliefs that a patient's history, rapport between patient and physician, and psychological preparation are of paramount importance. Pulos also states, "The healers are almost always in trance themselves using the "magnetic passes" (p. 207). It is easy to understand that when using hypnosis, the therapist must intently concentrate, exclude the surroundings, and focus on the patient's needs.

Fredericks (1966) pointed out the value of psychological preparation of patients prior to open heart surgery and used it routinely.

Esdaile was able to reduce postoperative mortality from infection from 50 to 5 percent. Antiseptics were unknown, as was the cause of frequently occurring infections. Cocke (1894) reported the use of hypnosis as the sole anesthetic in 42 minor and major operations. Ether was not introduced until 1846 and chloroform only in 1847.

The use of hypnosis as the sole anesthetic for major surgery is very dramatic but of limited use now. It was very important during World War II, because chemical anesthesia was not available at all times (Sampiman & Woodruff, 1946). There are many reports of the successful use of hypnosis since World War II. Mason (1955) did various types of surgery using hypnosis. Crasilneck, McCranie, and Jenkins (1956) described special indications of Hypnoanesthesia. Kroger (1957) used hypnosis for cesarean section and hysterectomy. Ruiz and Fernandez (1960) used hypnosis as an anesthetic in ophthalmology and Schwarcz (1965) reports on its use in urology. Bernstein (1965) presented three cases of successful use of hypnoanesthesia. Teitelbaum (1967) documented the effectiveness of hypnoanesthesia for major surgery and Patton (1969) used hypnosis for a thyroidectomy. Levitan (1978) reported the use of hypnosis as the sole anesthetic for abdominal surgery. Fredericks (1982) reported the use of hypnosis as an alternative method of anesthesia and pointed out all the advantages of this technique. Hilgard and Hilgard (1983) reviewed the use of hypnosis as the sole anesthetic and Morris, Nathan, Goebel, and Blass (1985) recommended the use of hypnosis for the morbidly obese. Kleinhauz and Eli (1993) pointed out that in dentistry, the use of hypnosis can play a major role. Levitan (1992) cited 27 surgical procedure with hypnosis as the sole anesthetic between 1977 and 1988, which was the beginning of his career as an oncologist. He did not encounter any postoperative wound infections and hypothesized that in the future, hypnoanesthsia would become more prevalent because of its safety, availability, and lack of infections. Unfortunately, this has not materialized, probably due to the many misconceptions which are still prevalent, even among physicians. Underdeveloped countries could benefit from its use, because they would not need expensive machines to deliver expensive anesthetic agents to perform necessary surgery.

There are several reports of patients using self-hypnosis for major surgery such as transurethral resection (Bowen, 1973) and cholecystectomy (Rausch, 1980). Thompson (1969) showed in a film the use of self-hypnosis for rhinoplasty and dermabrasion. This demonstrated her comfort and minimal loss of blood with this otherwise very bloody procedure. Kostka (1992) used self-hypnosis for two successive angioplasties, with good results and Hunter Farr (1997) has used self-hypnosis many times during her lifetime, the most recent one was for an emergency cesarean section. Botta (1999) reported self-hypnosis as anesthesia for liposuction surgery in great detail. There are several remarkable occurrences. First, that the surgeon was also the patient, second, that he did the surgery in the upright position, and last but not least, that his blood pressure was stable and he did not go into shock.

Because of the development, relative safety, and ease of administration of chemical anesthesia, hypnosis for major surgery is used rarely and only on special occasions, or upon the patient's request. Only about 10 to 20 percent of the population is thought to be capable of going deep enough to undergo major surgery. Hypnotic responsiveness, as well as motivation and expectations, play an important role. However, there are many advantages when using hypnosis rather than chemical anesthesia.

With hypnosis, it is possible to ameliorate or even prevent many problems we encounter with the use of chemical, local, or regional anesthesia:

1. Because of the absence of toxic effects from anesthetic agents, there is no depression of vital functions, such as the regulation of blood pressure, heart rate, regularity of the heart beat, etc. All reflexes and compensatory mechanisms are preserved. There is no depression of pulmonary function. The patient is able to swallow, cough, expectorate, and assume a comfortable position on the operating room table. Good position avoids nerve damage, which can be seen occasionally and which is caused by undue pressure or stretch of a nerve.

2. There is less blood loss during surgery because hypnotized patients can help their bodies to constrict blood vessels and shunt blood away from the operative site. Appropriate suggestions, which are made preoperatively, can be repeated intraoperatively when necessary. This has been observed by numerous surgeons: Clawson and Swade (1975) report two cases of massive hemorrhage which were stopped promptly with the use of hypnosis. Thompson (1969), in her film on rhinoplasty and dermabrasion, with the use of self-hypnosis, shows minimal loss of blood. Ralph August's film showing a cesarean

section under hypnosis loses hardly any blood, and Bennett (1986), whose well-controlled study was mentioned before, proved the value of such suggestions. What are these suggestions? To divert the flow of blood to other parts of the body and to constrict blood vessels in the operative area, by thinking and experiencing "cold, icy cold, like winter storms on the ocean."

3. All physiological functions return promptly, such as voiding, which eliminates the necessity of catheterization, and passing stool, even after hemorrhoidectomies (Bartlett, 1966; Doberneck, 1959; Hutchings, 1961). Patients become thirsty soon after surgery, thereby avoiding nausea and vomiting. They are able to take and retain fluids by mouth, decreasing the time during which they need intravenous hydration.

4. They need no premedication. In fact, narcotics are contraindicated because patients need to be wide awake and able to concentrate in order to follow suggestions, to dissociate, and deepen trance. They require less or no narcotics postoperatively (Benson, 1971; Wolfe, 1960), which avoids pulmonary complications, as well as nausea and vomiting.

5. More rapid wound healing has been reported, partially due to less edema (Van Dyke, 1970; Ewin, 1986, 1992; Enqvist et al., 1996). The thinking about and experiencing of warmth can actually increase blood flow to certain areas and promote healing by better oxygenation and increased transport of necessary elements for healing. On the other hand, in acute burns, the swelling can be prevented by concentrating on coolness and comfort.

6. As discussed previously, the decreased anxiety, stress, apprehension, and worry about losing consciousness with chemical anesthesia are very beneficial in many ways. The relaxation, transference, and interpersonal relationship between the patient and the surgeon or anesthesiologist are an integral part of the hypnotic experience. Looking forward to a successful completion of the surgery, with a discussion of postoperative activities and the implicit removal of fear of death, need to be accepted subconsciously by the patient.

7. Smoother and shortened postoperative rehabilitation and period of hospital stay (Egbert, 1964; Pearson, 1961) is important, especially in the present-day emphasis on cost containment.

8. Time distortion, which can easily be accomplished with the use of hypnosis, is very much appreciated by patients. The time required

for some surgery, which might take many hours, can be reduced considerably in the perception of the patient. Often, the first words spoken by the patient after the completion of the surgery are "Oh, is it over already?" Dissociation, distortion of perception and memory, as well as changes in mood are integral parts of the hypnotic experience.

9. Postoperative complications, such as pneumonia or atelectasis, can be prevented by the increased suggestibility, motivation, and willingness to follow suggestions to cough, move about, and frequently take deep breaths.

10. Extremely poor-risk patients and patients with contraindications to chemical or even local anesthesia can be hypnotized and thereby decrease the risk.

11. Severely injured patients arriving in the accident ward or the office of a private physician can be deeply hypnotized, even if they have never been hypnotized before. In these instances, motivation and expectancy on the part of the patient are very important, and many patients with average or even low hypnotic ability are able to get comfortable when hypnotic techniques are used.

12. The ingestion of a large meal prior to an accident will not delay the prompt surgery. When there is a contraindication to pump out the stomach, hypnosis can be used instead of chemical anesthesia.

13. Last but not least is the availability and the immediate capability to use hypnosis. There is no need for any equipment or device. The only requirement is the knowledge of the attending physician to help the injured or critically ill patient to go into hypnosis.

It is mandatory that the physician or psychologist using hypnosis in a particular emergency situation be well-trained and experienced in the use of hypnosis. Many injured people can even use self-hypnosis if they were exposed to hypnosis for any other reason in the past. Patients do not have to be transported to a hospital in a great hurry. If they are not in stable condition, and a fractured leg or arm can be immobilized on the spot, the transport can be made much less painful. Hypnosis was used extensively and with great success in the battlefields of the Second World War, which probably saved many lives.

Application

Hypnosis as the sole anesthetic can and has been used for any and all types of surgery. There are many reports in the literature. Some further examples are: Wolfe and Millet (1960), Hutchings (1961), Kolouch

(1962), Wollman (1964), Van Dyke (1970), Gruen (1972), Scott (1975), Lowenstein, Iwamoto and Schwartz (1981), Tucker and Virnelli (1985), Levitan & Harbaugh (1989), and Adams (1992).

One specific indication for the use of hypnosis is for neurosurgery, when it is imperative that the patient is awake and can respond to verbal commands. Anesthetics also interfere with the electroencephalogram, which needs to be used in certain types of brain surgery, as well as for research.

It seems that hypnotized patients are aware of pain at some unconscious level, even though they do not experience pain on a conscious level. They are comfortable, having developed analgesia in the target area. They can dissociate this discomfort from conscious experience. Hilgard (1973b) verified this with a subject using automatic writing and in 1975 introduced the metaphor of the "hidden observer" and tested its validity (Hilgard, Hilgard, Macdonald, Morgan & Johnson, 1978). The authors described the phenomenon by which a person registers and stores information in memory without being aware that the information has been processed (cited in Lynn, Mare, Kvaal, Segal, & Sivec, 1994). Watkins (1990, p. 1) postulates that "normal individuals, like multiple personalities and "hidden observer" subjects, can displace (dissociate) pain into "covert ego states." There is a difference between chemical analgesia and analgesia produced by hypnosis (Hilgard, 1978). Chemical analgesia is produced by chemical agents, while hypnotic analgesia is produced by the subject's own expectancy, imagination, imagery, dissociation, etc. It is not known what happens to the pain, which is possibly experienced by the hidden observer. Therefore one must weigh the advantages and disadvantages of both, chemical anesthesia and hypno-anesthesia. It seems that the advantages of the latter by far outweigh the disadvantages and more physicians should give patients the chance more often to avail themselves of this technique.

Implementation

It is important to take a detailed history, not only of the present problem but also of past experiences with surgery and anesthesia. Ego strength and general attitude towards life and adversities need to be determined. Is this a positive personality or a negative misanthrope? Misconceptions about hypnosis have to be removed and a discussion of possible alternatives should follow. Poor hypnotic responsiveness is not always a limiting factor in deciding whether or not to use hypnosis. However, when used as the sole anesthetic for elective surgery, it is important to evaluate hypnotic responsiveness with a simple and short regression technique. It would be ill advised to use hypnosis as the sole anesthetic with a patient who seems to be unable to go deep enough to dissociate, as well as create positive or negative hallucinations, a prerequisite for the development of analgesia or anesthesia. Many well-controlled studies, using immersion of one hand into ice water, have shown, that high susceptibles report significantly less pain and keep the anesthetized hand in ice water longer than low susceptibles (Hilgard, 1975a; Tennenbaum, Kurtz, & Bienias, 1990). Motivation and expectancy on the part of the patient are important for the development of analgesia. Prehypnotic explanations, attitudes, beliefs, and the development of rapport, as well as the induction process, modify expectancy. Kirsch (1994) found that expectancy plays a significant role in hypnotic inductions and their effects.

When doing research, it is important to determine the hypnotic ability of each subject in order to be able to make comparisons and establish significant differences between groups of subjects (Spiegel, 1989). Several excellent scales have been devised for testing hypnotizability prior to experimentation and they are used universally. Examples are the Stanford Scales (Weitzenhoffer & Hilgard, 1959, 1962), the Harvard Group Scale (Shor & Orne 1962), the Hypnotic Induction Profile (Spiegel, 1974; Spiegel & Spiegel, 1978). However, in clinical practice, these scales are less important, especially since a simple regression technique, combined with Spiegel's Eye-Roll (Spiegel, 1972), gives a good indication of the patient's hypnotic capability.

After developing rapport with the patient and answering all questions the patient might have, one may proceed to test the patient's hypnotic ability. This can be accomplished with a simple and short regression to an earlier age, to a classroom of the patient's choice, involving all senses and evaluating the patient's responses. We might ask the patient, in her own mind's eye, to draw a circle on the black board and to write her name, her first name and her last name into the circle. When this has been accomplished, we suggest she find an eraser and erase her name, followed by the question "what she can see on the black board now." Most patients are able to see some smudges and when questioned what exactly they wrote into the circle, most will recite their maiden name. This indicates that regression to an early age was successful, that the patient really felt that she was a child, in a classroom and obviously not married yet. If the patient is male, a single female, or she is married but kept her maiden name, one can ask whether the writing in the circle looks as they would sign a check today. In clinical practice, when not doing research, it is not important to determine the exact hypnotic capability of each patient, which would take additional time and possibly activate some resistance. Besides this, if patients cannot respond positively to some items of the scales, they might get discouraged, whereas with this very short regression technique, the patient is usually successful (Cheek, 1994). It is interesting to note that all patients contemplating surgery with hypnosis as the sole anesthetic tested as highs with this simple regression method. However, the majority of people fall into the moderate or low range of hypnotizability, when tested with various other scales (Pearson, 1973; Bates, 1993). One should not deprive patients of all the advantages that the use of hypnosis provides, as long as they prove to be able to develop analgesia.

It is of utmost importance that an anesthesiologist is either the administrator of hypnosis, or is in attendance and in charge of all other responsibilities, when the surgeon or some other practitioner initiates the hypnosis. There are several prerequisites for the successful execution of hypnosis for major surgery:

1. One must be well trained and skilled in the use of hypnosis. This only comes after training in an approved program and extensive use and practice. It would be inadvisable for a novice in the use of hypnosis to attempt to carry a patient through major surgery with hypnosis as the sole anesthetic. It also is imperative to have the proper equipment and availability to administer local, regional, or general anesthesia immediately, which might occur upon the patient's request, or in the judgment of the anesthesiologist or surgeon.

2. The patient should be a reasonably good subject. As mentioned before only about 10 to 20 percent of the general population are classified as high hypnotizables, with currently used scales. However, when the regression test was applied and these patients were able to dissociate, it was found that all patients were able to undergo major surgery with comfort. As mentioned previously, this is due to the fact that motivation, expectancy, and determination on the part of the patient play a very important role. It seems that the ability to dissociate is of critical importance as well. In emergencies, motivation far out-

weighs the measured hypnotizability of the patient and in such situations practically all patients respond favorably.

3. One must have compassion for patients' suffering, and protect them from guilt feelings in case they wish to have additional anesthesia. By all means, avoid a power struggle with the patient.

4. Both physician and patients must be convinced that they will be successful. Torem (1997) pointed out that physicians, using hypnosis, have to believe in its effectiveness. Any doubt or uncertainty on the physician's part would be counterproductive. In this very close relationship with patients, they are very much in tune with their caregivers and would perceive any hesitation on their part.

It is advisable to work closely with the surgical team and never to undermine the confidence the patient has in the surgeon and his or her skills. However, a discussion with surgeons to point out the possibility that patients will hear or perceive meaningful information at some level is very helpful (Cheek, 1959–1979; Halfen, 1986; Rossi & Cheek; 1988; and many others) (see Chapter 3). It is wise to caution them to exercise great care in discussing findings or prognosis in the presence of patients. Nathan, Morris, Goebel, and Blass (1987) reported the importance of this. It is interesting to note that information perceived during chemical anesthesia produces dense amnesia postoperatively. However, when hypnotized, regressed, and taken through the actual surgical experience, patients can vividly recall what was said and can exhibit severe stress and anxiety.

Procedure

If the regression test has been satisfactory, one might induce hypnosis with the use of Spiegel's eye-roll induction (Spiegel & Spiegel, 1978), followed by eye closure, followed by progressive relaxation and dissociation to a pleasant place of the patient's choice, or ask the patient to participate in a most enjoyable activity. Another example might be a technique, leading the patients into a castle, down the steps to a very special place, "their own private room." There they are safe and comfortable, and nothing can disturb them. In this castle, there are several levels with staircases connecting them. As they descend these staircases, they deepen hypnosis considerably. As the patients descend deeper and deeper, their level of dissociation deepens as well. This dissociation is often similar to an out of body experience. Patients really feel that they are physically there and involved in a specific role or activity (Campanella, 1993). Instead of taking the patient down, one can suggest the opposite and develop lightness and floating in a balloon. This has been described by Walsh (1976) and modified by Livnay (1996). Interestingly, suggestions of lightness have a paradoxically deepening effect on trance. Other deepening techniques could be sunsets, ocean waves, a waterfall, or other appropriate metaphors. After a few minutes of really enjoying and seeing, hearing, smelling, touching, and actually experiencing all the suggestions which are made, in addition to every thing else patients might experience, it is safe to assume that they are ready to develop analgesia.

At this time, patients should be taught ideomotor signaling (Cheek & LeCron, 1968; Rossi & Cheek, 1988; Hammond & Cheek, 1988), which is thought to be a way of reaching the unconscious. This seems to be a way to ascertain the readiness of the patient, as well as the successful execution of suggestions. The unconscious is described as part of the psyche, which can respond to questions in a very spontaneous way, without conscious thought. When, upon questioning, the response is positive, the finger "designated as the yes finger" will rise, and the development of glove anesthesia can be suggested. This is usually accomplished with the greatest of ease, because glove anesthesia can be developed in rather light stages of hypnosis, and one can assume that the patient is far beyond that point. One way to achieve glove anesthesia is to recall and recreate numbness, which the patient has experienced in the past during dental procedures, or to touch the patient's hand with a blunt object suggesting that a very powerful and rapidly acting local anesthetic is being injected. Zachariae and Bjerring (1994) demonstrated that pain report, as well as pain-related brain potentials, can be reduced by merely suggesting hypnotic analgesia. Another suggestion could be for the patient to go to a control room where all their sensations are stored. There is a rheostat which can be turned down, or even all the way off. They also might envision the hand enveloped in a big glove, made of thick padded leather, which protects the hand from any kind of injury and makes the hand insensitive to pain. To say "which protects the hand from any and all sensations" would be inaccurate, because patients do feel pressure and traction and it would be counterproductive to give patients the impression that they will not feel anything. Glove anesthesia is really a misnomer. It is glove analgesia and should be called such.

After showing the patient the difference between the analgesic hand

and the opposite hand, one can test the results by taking a sterile hypodermic needle, picking up a fold of skin on the analgesic dorsum and thrust the needle through the skin, so that both ends are visible. As a rule, there is no reaction on the part of the patient. When this has been accomplished, it is important to let patients open their eyes and actually see and feel how comfortable they are, with the needle protruding on both sides of the fold of the skin. This is very impressive to the patient. It is contrary to Barber's experience (1996) that the development of analgesia is difficult to achieve because it requires a positive hallucination of analgesia. In situations like this, the development of glove analgesia can be accomplished by almost all people who are motivated or simply curious to have the experience. All students in my course at the University of Pennsylvania, as well as volunteers in demonstrations during workshops, were able to accomplish glove analgesia. The difference might be that Barber suggests anesthesia in areas of pain, whereas the development of analgesia in areas of normal sensation, such as the dorsum of the hand, might be much easier to achieve.

The transference of the analgesia from the anesthetized hand to the operative area is not quite as easily accomplished. However, patients are very impressed when they see the hypodermic needle having pierced the skin of their hand, do not feel discomfort, and even may observe that, after the withdrawal of the hypodermic needle, only one specific area, either the entrance or the exit of the needle, bleeds. It seems that with motivation and dissociation this can be accomplished with relative ease. Another way to proceed would be to initiate a negative hallucination, teaching the patient to dissociate and regard the part of the body which needs the surgery to be absent, or not existing for the time of the surgery. This arm or leg can be hallucinated to the favorite place and involved in some absorbing activity. It is very important to limit this to the time of the surgery. It could be highly disturbing and threatening to the patient to lose part of the body without limitation of time. To tell patients that they will not feel anything is not only not true but also counter productive. The trust which has been developed might be lost. It is better to say: "You may feel what the surgeon is doing and possibly feel some pressure in the area, but you will be perfectly comfortable."

Prior to transferring the anesthesia to the operative site, a deepening technique should be used and the patient should be encouraged to go deeper and deeper relaxed and to enjoy all the pleasant sensations even more intently than previously. The transfer is accomplished by touching and rubbing the entire area with the anesthetized hand. This does not create any problem and can be accomplished in a very short time. After gently pricking the area with a pin, the success of the induced analgesia is tested, by applying an Allis clamp to the area of contemplated surgery and closing it to the second notch. A very careful observation of the patient's reaction will suggest the next step. Once again the patient will need to open her eyes and look at "that area." The surprise and the amazement which follows, seeing the instrument clamped on a fold in the skin and being perfectly comfortable, is very rewarding to the patient, as well as to the operator. The distortion of perception and apparently the lack of memory of previous experiences of pain is remarkable.

When working with patients in this fashion, it is not surprising to find oneself deeply involved with them. Transference and countertransference will be very obvious. The intense concentration necessary to achieve the desired results will lead to slipping into a state of altered awareness. This very strong transferential quality of the hypnotic experience, is probably responsible, to a great extent, for the successes in clinical practice. Scagnelli (1980) described rather vividly the use of hypnosis by the therapist as well as by the patient.

After encouraging the patient to close her eyes again and going deeper and deeper, one should try to elicit and discuss all the feelings the patient experienced up to that point. Patients are perfectly able to talk and remain in hypnosis. Their speech might be slower and their tone of voice lower than normal and they might lighten their level of hypnosis a bit, but they do not come out of trance unless there is an important reason for it. If this should happen, a very careful discussion and evaluation of the situation would be necessary. When patients react positively and describe their good feelings and there satisfaction with this experience, it is important to praise them and to encourage them, to be very proud of their success. Praise is very important. Neither the patient nor the practitioner knows how these astonishing results are achieved and patients need to be told that, whatever they are doing to produce these effects is exactly the right thing.

It is advisable to teach these patients self-hypnosis and have them practice the development of glove anesthesia and transference to the operative site several times a day, until the next visit. This can be accomplished by making a posthypnotic suggestion, explaining that since hypnosis is created by themselves, they can perform this exercise on their own. The value of this not only lies in the fact that with practice, patients become more proficient, but it also empowers them and increases their sense of control.

The taking of the history, clearing up all misconceptions, and teaching patients to enter hypnosis deep enough to produce analgesia in the operative area takes about one hour and can be accomplished with ease in most instances. When patients desire to undergo surgery with the use of hypnosis as their sole anesthetic, they engage physicians with the expectation of success, which facilitates the entire procedure.

The second and possibly a third visit should be used to teach the patient to transfer the anesthesia to the operative site by visualization instead of by actually touching the area. It is most astonishing how these patients can accomplish this in a very short time. Some patients, especially highly hypnotizables, are able to just turn off a switch and make the area insensitive to pain. It is important to teach patients to extend the anesthesia into the depth of the operative area so they may ignore all kinds of sensations, such as traction or the use of a cautery. These sensations are very different from an incision into the skin and patients need to be prepared for that. It can be accomplished by making appropriate suggestions of comparison to sensations, which the patient has experienced previously. Even the sound of the cautery has to be explained and incorporated into the experience. If this is not done, patients might get very uncomfortable and even feel pain. If that happens, all is not lost, as long as the physician is in control of the situation. Surgeons frequently use the cautery to stop oozing from tiny little blood vessels and patients have to be prepared for this sensation. Even the auditory perception of the buzzing of the instrument can make the patient uncomfortable. In such a situation, hypnosis has to be deepened by reinforcing previous suggestions, such as going back to their favorite place or activity and completely ignoring everything else. Having established good rapport and a trustworthy relationship with patients will facilitate this deepening process, and usually the patient will regain comfort easily. If this does not work promptly, it is mandatory to induce general anesthesia. Because an intravenous route has been established in the holding area prior to taking the patient into the operating room, it only takes a few seconds to accomplish this. If general anesthesia is contraindicated, the surgeon will either have to stop using the cautery or inject local anesthetics. To be able to deal with unexpected surgical procedures, as well as unexpected sensations, patients need to be made aware of such possibilities during the preoperative visit. Some patients are very much auditorily oriented and state that "When I practice, I can hear your voice." They will be helped a great deal by listening to a tape, made at one of their previous sessions. They should listen to the tape frequently, prior to surgery. This seems to make dissociation during surgery much easier.

This visit, to teach patients to go into trance and to develop analgesia in the operative area, takes no more than an hour and whether a third visit is advisable can be established during this encounter. Most of the time a third visit is not necessary. Schultz (1954) advocated taking patients through the surgical procedure during one of the preoperative visits. This seems not only unnecessary, but in many instances even contraindicated. Many patient's coping style is avoidance and they would react negatively to be informed about details of the operative procedure.

During the visit the night before surgery, when patients have been admitted to the hospital, they are asked to go into hypnosis on their own and appropriate suggestions are made, covering various topics, which were described in detail in Chapter 3. Such suggestions as the control of bleeding, the prompt return of all physiological functions, the lack of postoperative discomfort, and rapid wound healing should be included. This takes very little time and usually is successful because rapport has been established in previous visits and patients have been able to accomplish such astonishing control over their sensations. During surgery the anesthesiologist should converse freely with patients. Most of them enjoy the conversations and they will be helped by elaborating on details of the place and activity which they decided to hallucinate. Dissociation is very important and patients need to be able to accomplish it. These conversations should always be carried out in a very low voice, so as not to distract the surgeon. Only once did a surgeon tell me, after the completion of the surgery, that he was rather uncomfortable, making an incision on the patient's neck for a thyroidectomy, who was conscious and talking with me. We previously collaborated very successfully on a hysterectomy with hypnosis as the sole anesthetic. He told me this in a very friendly way and I could understand his feelings.

In the recovery room these patients are remarkable. They are tired, because they have done a tremendous amount of work, but they are relaxed and very proud of their accomplishment. The time spent with them in the recovery room is used to praise them and reinforce all the suggestions which were made preoperatively and in particular to stress the fact that all their physiological functions will return promptly and that they will feel thirsty and hungry very soon. This suggestion will prevent any nausea or vomiting. When they feel any sensation in the operative area, they should consider this as a sign that healing has begun already. The nurses are instructed not to put an emesis basin on their bed and not to ask them whether they have any pain. Patients are instructed to ask for the prescribed medication in case they should have some discomfort. However, the suggestion is made, since they were so comfortable during the surgery, they could be just as comfortable now.

In an emergency, patients need no preparation at all, other than for the surgeon or anesthesiologist to obtain the patient's trust and to establish rapport in a hurry. Hypnotic techniques can be used with great success. A patient weighing more than 200 pounds, with severe lobar pneumonia, high fever, and supposedly allergic to all local anesthetics was in active labor. General anesthesia was out of the question because of her pulmonary status, dyspnea, and high fever. She was a multipara, having had a Cesarean section for her last delivery. She now fell into active labor and arrived at the emergency room of a community hospital. There was the danger that she might rupture her uterus, if active contractions continued or increased. As far as her anesthesia was concerned, she had no prenatal instructions. The attending obstetrician had a serious problem on his hands. Luckily, he was well trained in the use of hypnosis, and after assuring the patient that he could carry her through the repeat section, with comfort and safety for her and her baby, she consented to cooperate with him as much as she possibly could. The obstetrician induced trance rapidly, continued to deepen hypnosis, by talking to her incessantly and making appropriate suggestions while he was scrubbing his hands. The patient was prepared for surgery by an assistant and the obstetrician continued to talk to her while performing the operation. She was comfortable throughout the entire surgery and was successfully delivered a healthy baby, by Cesarean section, with the use of hypnosis as the sole anesthetic.

It is interesting to note that, in cases of emergency, invariably patients seem to have a high hypnotic capacity. Is this just sheer luck? Or can the situation, the motivation and the expectancy influence the capability of the patient to go deep enough, to achieve the desired result?

The use of hypnosis as the sole anesthetic is of greatest value when emergencies arise and when there is no possibility to use general or regional anesthesia. When the patient chooses hypnosis, for whatever reason, or the attending surgeon or anesthesiologist decides that this is the best and safest way to undergo surgery, at this particular time and for this particular patient, hypnosis is of great value and usually can be achieved without problems. The prerequisites are (1) that the physician or other health care professional who helps the patient go into hypnosis deep enough to be comfortable, is well trained in the use of hypnosis, and (2) that the patient is interested in the experience and motivated to accomplish the desired goal.

James Esdaile (1846–1957), the British surgeon who used hypnosis as the sole anesthetic for major surgery many years ago, would be very interested and pleased to see the progress which has been made to avoid pain during surgery. He was a pioneer and credit must be given to him for his accomplishments. He also made us aware of the tremendous possibilities of using hypnosis for the treatment of pain in general, both acute and chronic. It is important to understand that, in general, hypnosis is not a treatment per se but, that its use gives leverage to each and every treatment modality. The exception is when it is used as the sole anesthetic in major surgery, when it seems to be the treatment per se.

REFERENCES

Adams, P.G. (1992). Liver biopsy under hypnosis. *Journal of Clinical Gastroenterology, 15,* 122–124.

Barber, J. (1996). Hypnosis and suggestion in the treatment of pain: A clinical guide. New York, London: W.W. Norton.

Bartlett, E.E. (1966). Polypharmacy versus hypnosis in surgical patients. *Pacific Medicine and Surgery, 74,* 109–112.

Bates, B.L. (1993). Individual differences in response to hypnosis. In J.W. Rhue, S.J. Lynn & I. Kirsch (Eds.), *Handbook of Clinical Hypnosis.* (pp 23–54). Washington, D.C.: American Psychological Association.

Bennett, H.L., Benson, D.R., & Kuiken, D.A. (1986). Preoperative instructions for decreased bleeding during spine surgery. *Anesthesiology, 65*(3A), A245.

Bensen, V.B. (1971). One Hundred cases of post-anesthetic suggestion in the recovery Room. *American Journal of Clinical Hypnosis, 14*(1) 9–15.

Bernstein, M.R. (1965). Significant value of hypnoanesthesia: Three clinical examples. *American Journal of Clinical Hypnosis 7*(3), 259–260.

Botta, S. A. (1998). Self-hypnosis as anesthesia for liposuction surgery. *American Journal of Clinical Hypnosis, 41*(4): 299–302.

Bowen, D.E. (1973). Transurethral resection under self-hypnosis. *American Journal of Clinical Hypnosis, 16*:132–134.

Campanella, G. (1993). Neurophysiologische Ueberlegungen zur Hypnose und deren moegliche Wirkungsweise bei kronischem Krebsschmerz. *Hypnose und Kognition 10,* 35–45.

Cheek, D.B., & LeCron, L. (1968). *Clinical hypnotherapy.* New York: Grune & Stratton.

Cheek, D.B. (1959). Subconscious perception of meaningful sounds during surgical anesthesia as reviewed under hypnosis. *American Journal of Clinical Hypnosis, 1*(3), 102–113.

Cheek, D.B. (1994). *Hypnosis: The application of ideomotor techniques.* Boston: Allyn & Bacon.

Clawson, T.A., Jr., & Swade, R.H. (1975). The hypnotic control of blood flow and pain: The cure of warts and the potential for the use of hypnosis in the treatment of cancer. *American Journal of Clinical Hypnosis, 17*(3),160–164.

Cocke, J.R., (1894). *Hypnotism.* Boston: Arena.

Crasilneck, H.B., McCranie, E.J., & Jenkins, M.T. (1956). Special indications for hypnosis as a method of anesthesia. *Journal of the American Medical Association. 126,* 1606–1608.

Doberneck, R.C., Griffen, W.O., Papermaster, A.A., Bonello, F., & Wagensteen, O.H. (1959). Hypnosis as an adjunct to surgical therapy. *Surgery, 46,* 299–304.

Egbert L. D., Battit G.E., Welch C.E., & Bartlett, M.K. (1964): Reduction of postoperative pain by encouragement and instruction of patients. *New England Journal of Medicine, 270*(16), 825–827.

Enqvist, B., Konow, L., & Bystedt, H. (1996). Stress reduction, preoperative hypnosis and perioperative suggestion in maxillo-facial surgery: Somatic responses and recovery. *Hypnosis, 23*(2), 76–82.

Esdaile, J. (1846). *Mesmerism in India and its practical applications in surgery and medicine.* London: Longmans, Brown, Green and Longmans. As quoted in Gravitz, 1988.

Ewin, D.M. (1986b). Emergency room hypnosis for the burned patient. *American Journal of Clinical Hypnosis, 29*(2), 115–118.

Ewin, D.M. (1992b). The use of hypnosis in the treatment of burn patients. *Psychiatric Medicine, Vol. 10*(4), 79–87.

Fredericks, L.E. (1966). Anesthesia for open heart surgery. Springfield, IL: Charles C Thomas.

Fredericks, L.E. (1982). Alternate methods of anesthesia. *Dangerous properties of industrial materials report, 2*(4), 6–15.

Gravitz, M.A., (1988): Early uses of hypnosis as surgical anesthesia. *American Journal of Clinical Hypnosis, 30*(3), 201–208.

Gruen, W. (1972). A successful application of systematic self-relaxation and self-suggestions about postoperative reactions in a case of cardiac surgery. *International Journal of Clinical and Experimental Hypnosis, 20*(3), 143–151.

Halfen, D. (1986). What do "anesthetized patients" hear? *Anesthesiology News,* March 12, p12.

Hammond, D.C., & Cheek, D.B. (1988). Ideomotor signaling: A method for rapid unconscious exploration. In D.C. Hammond (Ed.), *Hypnotic induction & suggestion.* Des Plaines, IL: American Society of Clinical Hypnosis Press, 90–97.

Hilgard, E. R., Morgan, A. H., & McDonald, H. (1975a). Pain and dissociation in the cold pressor test: A study of hypnotic analgesia with hidden reports through automatic key-pressing and automatic talking. *Journal of Abnormal Psychology, 84:* 280–289.

Hilgard, E. R., & Hilgard, J. R. (1983). Hypnosis in the relief of pain. Los Altos, CA: William Kaufman, pp120–143.

Hilgard, E. R. (1973b). The domain of hypnosis. *American Psychologist, 28,* 972–982.

Hilgard, E. R., Hilgard, J., Macdonald, H., Morgan, A.H., & Johnson, L.S. (1978). Covert pain in hypnotic analgesia: Its reality as tested by the real-simulator design. *Journal of Abnormal Psychology, 87,* 655–663.

Hunter Farr, J. (1997). Self-hypnosis during a cesarean section. 14th International Congress of Hypnosis, San Diego, CA.

Hutchings, D. (1961). The value of suggestions given under anesthesia: A report and evaluation of 200 consecutive cases. *American Journal of Clinical Hypnosis 4*(1), 26–29.

Kihlstrom, J.F., & Schachter, D.L. (1990). Anesthesia, amnesia and the cognitive unconscious. In B. Bonke, W. Fitch, & K. Millar (Eds.), *Memory and awareness in anaesthesia.* Amsterdam: Swets & Zeitlinger, pp 21–44.

Kirsch, I. (1994). Clinical hypnosis as a non-deceptive placebo: Empirically derived techniques. *American Journal of Clinical Hypnosis, 37*(2), 95–106.

Kleinhauz, M., & Eli, I. (1993). When Pharmacological anesthesia is precluded: The Value of hypnosis as the sole anesthetic agent in dentistry. *Special Care Dentists, 13*(1), 15–18.

Kolouch, F.T. (1962). Role of suggestion in surgical convalescence. *Archives of Surgery, 85,* 304–315.

Kostka, M. (1992). Personal experience with "Use of hypnosis berfore and during angioplasty." Letter to the Editor. *American Journal of Clinical Hypnosis, 34*(4), 281–282.

Kroger, W.S., & DeLee, S.T. (1957). Hypnoanesthesia for cesarean section and hysterectomy. *Journal of the American Medical Association, 163,* 442–444.

Levitan, A.A., & Harbourgh, T.E. (1989). Hypnoanalgesia and hypnotizability. *Hypnosis, 16*(3), 140–148.

Levitan, A.A. & Harbourgh, T.E. (1992). Hypnotizability and Hypnoanalgesia: Hypnotizability of patients using hypnoanalgesia during surgery. *American Journal of Clinical Hypnosis, 34*(4), 223–226.

Levitan, A.A. (1978). Use of hypnosis as sole anesthesia for abdominal surgery. Presented at the Annual Meeting of the Society for Clinical and Experimental

Hypnosis. Ashville, N.C.

Livnay, S., (1996). Is hypnosis full of hot air? The Utilization of a hot air balloon imaginal technique (H.A.B.I.T.). *Hypnosis 23*(3), 137–143.

Lowenstein, L.N., Iwamoto, K., & Schwartz, H. (1981). Hypnosis in high risk ophthalmological patients. *Ophthalmic Surgery, 12,* 34–41.

Lynn S.J., Mare, C., Kvaal, S., Segal, D., & Sivec, H. (1994). The hidden observer, hypnotic dreams, and age regression: Clinical Implications. *American Journal of Clinical Hypnosis, 37*(2), 130–142.

Mason, A.A. (1955). Surgery under hypnosis. *Anesthesia, 10,* 295–299.

Morris, D.M., Nathan, M.G., Goebel, R.A., & Blass, M.H. (1985). Hypnoanesthesia in the morbidly obese. *Journal American Medical Society, 253*(22), 3292–3295.

Nathan, R., Morris, D., Goebel, R.A., & Blass, N. (1987). Preoperative and intraoperative rehearsal in hypnoanesthesia for major surgery. *American Journal of Clinical Hypnosis, 29,* 238–241.

Patton, I.B. (1969). Report on thyroidectomy performed under hypnosis. *Journal of the Medical Association of Alabama, 38,* 617–619.

Pearson, R. E. (1961). Response to suggestions given during general anesthesia. *American Journal of Clinical Hypnosis, 4*(2): 106–114.

Pearson, R.E. (1973). Lecture given at the Institute of the Pennsylvania Hospital, Philadelphia, PA., February, 1973.

Pulos, L. (1980). Mesmerism revisited: The effectiveness of Esdaile's techniques in the production of deep hypnosis and total body hypnoanaesthesia. *American Journal of Clinical Hypnosis, 22*(4), 206–211.

Rausch, V. (1980). Cholecystectomy with self-hypnosis. *American Journal of Clinical Hypnosis, 22*(3), 124–129.

Rossi, E.L., & Cheek, D.B. (1988). *Mind-body therapy: Ideodynamic healing in hypnosis.* New York: W.W. Norton.

Ruiz, O.R., & Fernandez, A. (1960). Hypnosis as an anesthetic in ophthalmology. *American Journal of Ophthalmology, 50,* p 163.

Sampiman, R., & Woodruff, M. (1946). Some observations concerning the use of hypnosis as a substitute for anesthesia. *Medical Journal of Australia, 1,* 393.

Scagnelli, J. (1980). Hypnotherapy with psychotic and borderline patient: The use of trance by patient and therapist. *American Journal of Clinical Hypnosis, 22*(3), 164–169.

Schultz, J. (1954). Some remarks about the techniques of hypnosis as an anesthetic. *British Journal of Medical Hypnotism, 5,* 23–25.

Schwarcz, B.E. (1965). Hypnoanalgesia and hypnoanesthesia in urology. *Surgical Clinics of North America, 45,* 1547–1555.

Scott, D.L. (1975). Hypnoanalgesia for major surgery. A psychodynamic process. *American Journal of Clinical Hypnosis, 16*(2), 84–91.

Shor, R.E., & Orne, E.C. (1962). *Harvard group scale of hypnotic susceptibility, Form A.,* Palo Alto, CA: Consulting Psychologists Press.

Spiegel, H. (1989): Should therapists test for hypnotizability? *American Journal of Clinical Hypnosis, 32,* 15–16.

Spiegel, H., & Spiegel D. (1978). *Trance and Treatment: Clinical Uses of Hypnosis.* New

York: Basic Books.

Spiegel, H., (1974). *Manual for hypnotic induction profile.* New York: Soni Medica, Inc.

Spiegel, H., (1972). An eye-roll test for hypnotizability. *Amerian Journal of Clinical Hypnosis, 15*(1), 25–28.

Tennenbaum, S.J., Kurtz, R., & Bienias, J.L. (1990). Hypnotic susceptibility and experimental pain reduction. *American Journal of Clinical Hypnosis, 33*(1), 40.

Thompson, K. (1969). *Rhinoplasty and dermabrasion under hypnosis.* Motion Picture Film Services, Inc. 209 Ninth Street, Pittsburg, PA.

Teitelbaum, M. (1967). Hypnosis in surgery and anesthesiology. *Anesthesia and Analgesia, 46*(5), 509–514.

Torem, M.S. (1997). Pharmacotherapy augmented by hypnosis. Workshop, The 14th International Congress of Hypnosis. San Diego, CA.

Tucker, K.R. (1985). The use of hypnosis as a tool in plastic surgery. *Plastic Reconstructive Surgery, 76*(1),140–146.

Van Dyke, P.B. (1970). Some uses of hypnosis in the management of the surgical patient. *American Journal of Clinical Hypnosis, 12*(4), 227–235.

Walsh, S.L. (1976). The red balloon technique of hypnotherapy. A clinical note. *International Journal of Clinical and Experimental Hypnosis, 24*(1), 10–12.

Watkins, J.G., & Watkins, H.H. (1990). Dissociation and displacement: Where goes the "ouch?". *American Journal of Clinical Hypnosis, 33*(1), 1–10.

Weitzenhoffer, A. M., & Hilgard, E.R. (1959). *Stanford susceptibility scale, Forms A and B.* Palo Alto, CA: Consulting Psychologists Press.

Weitzenhoffer, A.M., & Hilgard, E.R. (1962). *Stanford hypnotic susceptibility scale, Form C.* Palo Alto, CA: Consulting Psychologists Press.

Wolfe L., & Millet J. (1960). Control of postoperative pain by suggestion under general anesthesia. *American Journal of Clinical Hypnosis, 3*(2), 109–112.

Wollman, L. (1964). Hypnosis for the surgical patient. *American Journal of Clinical Hypnosis, 7,* 83–85.

Zachariae R., & Bjerring, P. (1994). Laser-induced pain-related brain potentials and sensory brain potentials in high and low hypnotizable subjects during hypnotic suggestions of relaxation, dissociated imagery, focused analgesia, and placebo. *The International Journal of Clinical and Experimental Hypnosis, 42*(1), 56–79.

Chapter 6

HYPNOSIS IN THE INTENSIVE CARE UNIT

Lillian E. Fredericks

Most patients in the intensive care unit are post major surgery, usually awake and responsive to verbal commands, or else comatose patients who are unresponsive.

Patients who can respond to verbal commands and who can make their wishes known can be dealt with easily, whether they were prepared with hypnosis preoperatively or not. However, patients who were prepared with hypnotic techniques show a great deal of difference in their requirements for narcotics, their response to verbal requests such as to take a few deep breaths, the absence of nausea and vomiting, the ability to empty their bladder when it is full, the prompt reappearance of intestinal motility, and their state of relaxation and comfort as compared to patients who were unprepared. These patients tolerate the presence of an endotracheal tube and the respirator well, because they were informed prior to surgery of the purpose and the importance of the function of these appliances. They are not concerned if they are receiving a transfusion, because they were told if the necessity arises, blood will be administered. Under these circumstances, it is important to make sure that patients understand that this does not mean that they were unsuccessful in following our suggestions, but that this was unforeseen and it would not have been wise to withhold blood. It is important to avoid any guilt feelings patients might develop when they see that things have changed in some way. All in all, these patients can be classified as patients who stabilize promptly and progress according to expectations. Talking to these patients for a few minutes, praising them, telling them how well they have done and answering any questions they may have, will remind them that surgery has been completed and that they can feel quite comfortable. Frequently, they inquire how soon they can go back to their rooms to see their families. If they are stable, they can be transferred as soon as their surgeon allows it. Nurses are instructed not to put an emesis basin next to these patients and never to ask them whether they feel sick at their stomach or have any pain. They are to administer sedation or analgesics only when the patient requests it. Usually these patients will only request medication when they experience pain which they cannot control with self-hypnosis, which they have learned preoperatively.

Unconscious patients require a great deal of attention. Unconsciousness or coma can have many different causes, including chemical anesthesia, severe trauma, cerebrovascular accident, or narcotic overdose. These conditions have in common that the patient cannot verbally respond when spoken to. Anesthesiologists usually get involved with these patients when they arrive in the operating room, or in the intensive care unit, when the acute phase of their treatment has been taken care of. Even though they seem to be unresponsive to verbal command, it should be possible to communicate with them on hypnotic levels. As mentioned in a previous chapter, critically ill, severely injured, hemorrhaging, and comatose patients often are in a state of altered consciousness and increased suggestibility. Weitzenhoffer (1996 p. 318) lists eight signs of hypnosis which bear some mention, other than catalepsy, and one can observe many of these signs in comatose patients. They also are vulnerable to indirect suggestions and to misinterpretation of innocent remarks and conversations. They need to be protected from psychological trauma, and this state of heightened suggestibility should be used to their advantage. It is important to attempt to communicate with these patients, because they often perceive meaningful information. Kihlstrom (1980) states that information processing also goes on in sleep and deep chemical anesthesia. Many Russian experimentors showed that learning during sleep is possible. Patients can be affected positively or negatively by the information they receive without conscious perception.

There is overwhelming evidence and a vast body of literature documenting that patients perceive and encode meaningful sensory perceptual information even in deep planes of surgical anesthesia (Cheek, 1959, 1964, 1959–1979; Levinson, 1965; Scott, 1972; Guerra, 1980; Bennett, 1988; Peebles, 1989). Some investigators who used numbers, letters, unrelated words, or irrevelant sentenses in their experiments reported negative results (Trustman, 1977; Millar, 1983; Eich, 1984, 1985). There seems to be a difference in perception and encoding of meaningful information versus irrelevant numbers, letters, sentences, or words. Postoperative questioning for memories is negative. But, when these patients are regressed in hypnosis to the operative experience and ideomotor signals are used, one can get a great deal of information (Rossi & Cheek, 1988, p. 21). Surgical anesthesia apparently blocks conscious, declarative verbal memory. When hypnotized and accessed on a nonverbal, behavioral level, such as pulling on an ear, verbal memories are accessed with ideomotor signaling (Bennett, 1984, 1985). Consciousness is not necessary for hearing and imprinting of sounds. Words can be perceived and can cause a response on an unconscious level, without conscious awareness (Kihlstrom, 1980). Encoding of meaningful sensory information occurs not only during sleep and surgical anesthesia but also in comatose and critically ill patients (Rossi & Cheek, 1988 p.186). Such information apparently is stored in a form which is split off, dissociated from consciousness, and not accessible to conscious awareness, except with the use of hypnotic interventions. The fact that it was shown that subjects during natural sleep are able to perceive and remember spoken material (Hoskovec, 1966) led us to hypothesize that comatose patients also can perceive meaningful information. The fact that these patients are unresponsive does not necessarily mean that their auditory as well as other receptive organs are not functioning. These patients have been shown to be aware of the meaning of words as well as touch (Cheek, 1994 p. 253). Since comatose patients can be reached verbally, hypnotic techniques are helpful in many ways. Crasilneck (1962) reported that eight out of ten patients, dying of cancer, continued their response to a hypnotic command, to touch the thumb and fourth finger of one hand, even though they revealed no other evidence of interaction with the environment and were considered clinically unconscious. Furthermore, a medical student on call apparently was able to communicate with a patient who was considered unconscious (Borrows, 1983) and Johnson (1987) used hypnotic techniques successfully with a woman who had been comatose for more than four months. Johnson's conclusion was that hypnotic techniques may be valuable in reaching, comforting, or stimulating the patient and/or facilitating the healing of some individuals in coma.

Procedure

We worked with several comatose patients. Most of whom had sustained severe trauma. The rationale of using hypnotic techniques was that we believed that suggestions of relaxation and vivid imagery, as well as dissociation to a pleasant place could increase comfort, especially when patients needed repeated injections or needed to undergo painful procedures. We assumed that if patients could hear, if they could subconsciously accept our suggestions, we could not only make them more comfortable but also influence their physiological functions, healing powers, and immune systems. We were encouraged by the fact that a great deal of research had been done during the past years to show that appropriate suggestions under hypnosis can influence and alter physiological parameters. Hall (1983), among others, suggested that hypnosis may potentially be able to alter immune responses in order to influence the underlying biochemical factors of physical disease.

During many years of practice in a large community hospital and later in a university hospital, we frequently visited comatose patients in the emergency room and in the intensive care unit. Some of them had been unconscious for several days, some only for a few hours. We saw them at least once a day, preferably twice, in the early morning and late in the afternoon. When dealing with patients whose eyes were open, usually glazed and with a blank stare without focusing, an eye fixation induction technique using some bright object such as a silvery pen was used. After several attempts and a great deal of patience, at times one could see at least a noticeable attempt at eye closure. When this did not occur, a gentle closing of their eyelids with one's fingers, while continuing to talk to them was indicated. If upon arrival the patient's eyes were closed, we felt it was important to greet the patient and to talk to him or her, always addressing by the first name. An introduction would follow explaining the purpose of our visit. The maintenance of bodily contact with the patient's hand or arm seemed important because it added extraverbal communication which helps. At times, the pulse rate would vary according to the type of suggestions which were made. When working with such patients repeatedly, some definite signs can occur which show that they were reached at some level. At times, one can observe some motion in their arms or legs, or even the mouth can move as though the patient attempted to talk. One comatose patient squeezed my hand upon request, after I had worked with her for a week. When using hypnosis there is a reciprocal influence by the hypnotist upon the patient and by the patient on the hypnotist. This interaction, the empathy, the influence of one upon the other can be observed at times.

For obvious reasons, which were explained in Chapter 3, the word "hypnosis" is never used. Talking to comatose patients about comfort, relaxation, hope, and determination to get well always using vivid imagery, trying to have them visualize various places, such as their own home, sitting in front of their television, enjoying a most interesting and stimulating movie, seems to be most appropriate since such dissociation is known to be very successful with surgical patients. The suggestion to go to a beach of their choice, or up into a mountain area can be used as well. The suggestions "not only see the beauty of the place, but also hear some familiar sounds, smell some flowers, touch familiar objects, and really feel that you are there and enjoy it to the fullest" seem to show a response at times. It is important to make it relevant and appropriate to the patient's age and circumstances. This can be obtained from studying the chart in advance. Sometimes this is rather difficult, because some histories are short and not detailed, often provided by a relative or friend rather than by the patient. It is important to inform these patients that they are in a safe place, that they are well taken care of and that they could be relaxed and comfortable at all times. Specific suggestions, to promote healing, to increase physical strength and alertness as well as continuous positive thinking should be made. To suggest imagining all the nice things they will be able to do in the future when they are back home again and in good health might be helpful as well. All these suggestions must be relevant and appropriate according to the pathology at hand.

If they can perceive messages, they might be able to use self-hypnosis to their advantage and one might suggest that they may create this wonderfully relaxing and comfortable state all on their own. This would help their body to rejuvenate and make it function again as it did in previous times. All they needed to do is imagine, in their own mind's eye, that they are in their favorite place, doing whatever they love to do, and to rehearse all the suggestions they were given. The more frequently they would do this little exercise (self-hypnosis), the better they would feel. In this way, they also could hasten their recovery.

One half hour talking to each patient seems to be appropriate. The suggestions should always be positive given in a soft voice, confident and hopeful. It is unfortunate that, as a rule, these patients can only be followed for such a short time, until they are discharged from the hospital to a longtime healthcare facility, or until they die. It might be possible to see more encouraging results if they could be treated for a longer period of time.

Since this is only a clinical report of experiences, over many years of practicing hypnosis and hypnotic techniques in an active hospital environment, we can only present impressions and hope that they will stimulate interest and lead to well-documented clinical research. This should be possible in any hospital which has an emergency room and intensive care unit as well as in a healthcare facility caring for comatose patients.

REFERENCES

Bennett, H.L., & Davis, H.S. (1984). Nonverbal response to intraoperative conversation. *Anesthesia and Analgesia, 63:*185.

Bennett, H.L. (1988). Perception and memory for events during adequate general anesthesia for surgical operation. In H.M. Pettinati (Ed.), *Hypnosis and memory.* New York: Guilford, pp. 193–231.

Bennett, H.L., Davis, H.S., & Giannini, J.A. (1985). Non-verbal response to intraoperative conversation. *British Journal of Anaesthesia, 57*(2), 174–179.

Borrows, A. (1983). A medical student on call. *Journal of the American Medical Association, 249*(9), 1128.

Cheek, D.B. (1959). Subconscious perception of meaningful sounds during surgical anesthesia as reviewed under hypnosis. *American Journal of Clinical Hypnosis, 1*(3), 102–113.

Cheek, D.B. (1959–1979). Awareness of meaningful sounds under general anesthesia: Considerations and a review of the literature. In H.J. Wain (Ed.), *Theoretical and clinical aspects of hypnosis,* 1981, p 87. Miami, FL: Symposia Specialists.

Cheek, D.B. (1964). Further evidence of persistence of hearing under chemo-anesthesia: Detailed case report. *American Journal of Clinical Hypnosis, 7*(1), 55–59.

Cheek, D.B. (1994). *Hypnosis: The application of ideomotor techniques.* Boston: Allyn & Bacon.

Crasilneck, Harold B. (1962). Some empirical findings associated with hypnosis. In Kline, Milton V. (Ed.), *The nature of hypnosis.* New York: Institute of Research in Hypnosis.

Eich, E. (1984). Memory for unattended events: Remembering with and without awareness. *Memory and Cognition, 12*(2), 105–111.

Eich, E. (1985). Anesthesia, amnesia, and the memory/awareness distinction. *Anesthesia Analgesia, 64*(12), 1143–1148.

Guerrra, F. (1980). Awareness under general anesthesia. In F. Guerra & J.A. Aldrete (Eds.), *Emotional and psychological responses to anesthesia and surgery.* New York: Grune & Stratton, pp. 1–8.

Hall, H.H. (1983). Hypnosis and the immune system: A review with implications for cancer and the physiology of healing. *American Journal of Cinical Hypnosis, 25,* 92–103.

Hosover, J. (1966). Hypnopedia in the Soviet Union: A critical review of recent major experiments. *International Journal of Clinical and Experimental Hypnosis, 14:*308–315.

Johnson, G.M. (1987). Hypnotic imagery and suggestion as an adjunctive treatment in a case of coma. *American Journal of Clinical Hypnosis. 29*(4), 255–259.

Kihlstrom, J.F., Evans, F.G., Orne, E.C., & Orne, M.T. (1980). Attempting to breach post hypnotic amnesia. *Journal of Abnormal Psychology, 89*(5) 603–616.

Levinson, B.W. (1965). States of awareness under general anesthesia. *British Journal of Anaesthesiology, 37,* 544–546.

Millar, K. (1983). Recognition of words presented during general anaesthesia. *Ergonomics, 26*(6), 585–594.

Peebles, M.J. (1989). Through a glass darkly: The psychoanalytic use of hypnosis with post-traumatic stress disorder. *The International Journal of Clinical and Experimental Hypnosis, 37*(3), 192–206.

Rossi, E.L., & Cheek, D.B. (1988). *Mind-body therapy: Ideodynamic healing in hypnosis.* New York: W.W. Norton.

Scott, D.L. (1972). Awareness during general anesthesia. *Canadian Anaesthesia Society Journal, 19,* 173–183.

Trustman, R., Dubovsky, S., & Titley, R. (1977). Auditory perception during general anesthesia – myth or fact? *International Journal of Clinical and Experimental Hypnosis, 25*(2), 88–105.

Weitzenhoffer, A.M. (1996). Catalepsy tests: What do they tell us? *Amerian Journal of Clinical and Experimental Hypnosis: 44*(4), 307–322.

Chapter 7

HYPNOSIS IN THE EMERGENCY ROOM

LILLIAN E. FREDERICKS

The emergency room usually is a very busy place and when several patients are brought in at the same time, triage is necessary. Even though time is very precious, one must take a quick history and physical examination in order to evaluate the patient and make a proper diagnosis. As a rule, patients will have been admitted by a nurse, intern, or resident whose notes will have documented some valuable information and thereby save time. Much harm could be done if an incorrect diagnosis were made. Hypnotic techniques are powerful tools and suggestions need to be specific and appropriate, according to the problems at hand.

As noted in the Chapter 3, severely injured, frightened, hemorrhaging, shocked, critically ill, unconscious, or comatose patients can be considered to be in a state of altered awareness. They are very vulnerable and in a state of heightened suggestibility due to the illness or injury and the increased anxiety, fear, apprehension, and arousal which accompany such an event (Cheek, 1969). It is essential to realize that an anxious voice or negative comments made by caregivers or even friends or family may have a detrimental effect. In this altered state, patients focus their attention on the caregiver and to a great extent exclude their surroundings. These people often take words and sentences literally, and may interpret them in a childlike manner. They seem to be emotionally regressed. In acute emergencies, the power of reason, the critical thinking mind is not used. It is apparently subjugated to a phylogenetically older, more primitive, more spontaneous mode of functioning. Since people in authority exert a tremendous influence upon patients in this altered state, careless conversations can be misinterpreted and have detrimental effects. Negative suggestions, such as "You will not feel any pain," may be interpreted by the patient as "I will be dead and therefore cannot feel any pain" or that the contemplated procedure must include painful maneuvers. Nonverbal communications, such as hesitation, a sigh, or an anxious look, can also be misinterpreted by these patients. Physicians as well as all other health care professionals must be cognizant of this and choose words carefully. It is appropriate to suggest that patients ignore any sounds they hear except when addressed by name. Patients must be informed about the fact that we are experienced specialists, and that we will do everything in our power to help them and make them comfortable and safe. In conversations, explaining what will be done and telling them that they too can help their bodies to stabilize and heal, they will be distracted and unlikely to concentrate on their injuries. Simple goals such as "your body knows how to stop this bleeding, but you can help it by making the area of your injury cold and comfortable" should be established, and in doing so, possibly stop the processes leading to shock (Rossi & Cheek, 1988 p. 185).

How does one recognize spontaneously occurring hypnosis? When a patient's eyes are open, they have a glazed look, without focusing, and their facial expression is flat. Frequently, one can observe fluttering eyelids and notice an economy of action, muscular activity which is slowed or absent, tone of voice is low, and speech is slow and usually rather subdued. Their behavior and their understanding is childlike and literal (Cheek, 1994). When the patient is asked: "Would you mind telling me your name?" in many cases, the answer would be "No" (i.e., "I wouldn't mind"). When asked "Please tell me your name," the patient will tell his or her name.

Since these patients are in a state of altered awareness, it is possible to talk to them much the same, as though hypnosis had been induced formally. Appropriate suggestions can be made immediately without any hesitation. However, the physician must feel confident that hypnosis will offer them the possibility to improve their physiological as well as psychological malfunctions, speed their power of healing, and often improve their chance of survival. This conviction and enthusiasm is imparted to the patient and frequently incredible results are seen. Patients get unconsciously motivated to use all their resources, which seems to activate their immune and endocrine systems and the production of antibodies (Smith, 1995; Olness, 1997). Emergencies activate the highest degree of responsivity.

It is important to collect one's thoughts carefully before approaching these patients. In order to transmit confidence and hope to these patients, the physician needs to be inperturbable (Osler, 1932). Conscious as well as unconscious patients are very perceptive and will react to the demeanor, attitude, and competence of the caregiver. Even the tone of voice can make a difference.

If patients are conscious, it is wise to acknowledge that we understand that they are hurting but that we will help them to be comfortable and safe. Such reassurances will help them to relax. At first, one may solicit their help and engage them in our activities. It is useful to get a commitment from them to leave the job to us, since we are in charge right now and have been trained to take care of patients " just like you." Later, one should help them to dissociate to a pleasant place of their choice or involve them in conversations about their children or family, etc. This distraction technique helps a great deal and allows them to concentrate on pleasant feelings, rather than on their pain and suffering. Talking about the good things of this particular situation, such as "only one bone is fractured or only one part of the body has been burned," will also have a calming influence. To focus on present needs and on the future rather than on the past and all the terrible things which have happened will increase their expectancy of success. Kleinhaus and Solomon (1995) used time progression, among other hypnotherapeutic techniques, with soldiers who suffered from combat stress reactions and described good results with these strategies.

Testing for hypnotizability is not necessary in situations like this. Motivation is far more important than the hypnotic capability of the patient. Furthermore, if the patient does not do well on some of the test items of the scales, it may be discouraging and counterproductive. It also is time consuming and in many situations, loss of time may be detrimental.

In the beginning, one should tell patients the plan of action on their level of understanding. This will engage them and make them part of the team. It not only distracts them but also empowers them and makes it more interesting for them. They are less likely to concentrate on their pain and misery. All of this can be done while attending to their physical needs. Since they are in an altered state of awareness, one should talk slowly in a relaxed way, making appropriate pauses, so patients can let it sink in and follow specific suggestions and instructions. It is important to make only positive suggestions, because positive suggestions are accepted more readily than negative suggestions, and to avoid misinterpretations, which might have a negative effect. Such suggestions might be: "Your body really knows what needs to be done to make these muscles soft and comfortable, but you can help it by taking a nice deep breath, and as you exhale, just let it go." For patients with asthma to "relax all the tiny muscles in the walls of your breathing tubes and you can help it by letting your mind think of happy times, when you were at your best, felt well, and were doing something you really love to do. Your body and mind work together and your healing powers will be greatly augmented when you are relaxed and at peace with yourself and the world." When a patient has been involved in an accident, this often results in anger or guilt, depending upon the patient's interpretation of the cause of the accident. If patients think that they caused the accident, guilt feelings may be overwhelming, and if the cause of the accident was deemed to be the other person's fault, anger and rage may prevail. Some patients express their rage or disappointment very early and it is good to help such patients to deal with these emotions appropriately, even at this early stage.

More specific explanations need to be given when dealing with more intelligent patients, explaining the physiological reactions of the body to injuries, how the body functions to heal the injured organs and tissues, and how they can help their bodies by visualizing these sequences. When patients are in severe pain, it is good to talk about the conduction of the sensation of pain from the periphery where the injury happens to be, via certain nerves to the central nervous system, just like electricity travels through wires to a light bulb or some other end station. It is useful to explain that only when the sensation reaches the cortex of the brain will the pain be perceived as such. It is possible for them to interrupt this transmission along the way, or they can use a rheostat to turn it down or even switch it off completely. There are two components to the experience of severe pain. One is the somatic component, the actual physical impact, and the other is the psychic experience, the interpretation, the perception, and the specific meaning of the pain. Hypnosis and hypnotic techniques are very powerful tools to decrease, or even eliminate, the psychological components which usually are the more important ones.

Since motivation is more important than depth of trance, deepening spontaneously occurring hypnosis is not necessary. These patients are very anxious to get relief from suffering, and thereby hypnotic interventions are usually very successful.

In general, a permissive hypnotic approach is advisable, but in emergencies, an in-control, confident approach is more helpful. First, one needs to get the attention of the patient, and at the same time narrow the focus of attention to the therapist's voice and suggestions. Next, helping them to dissociate, to turn inward and really experience our suggestions of seeing and hearing and feeling is important. This can be accomplished by suggesting that, in their mind's eye, they should go to their favorite place, watching all the details and truly feel that they are there. They might want to be involved in a chosen activity, like swimming or playing baseball or any other activity which seems desirable. Patients can communicate with us without coming out of hypnosis and one can initiate an all engrossing conversation. Under these circumstances, patients can be completely involved in the focus of their choice and be oblivious to any procedure being performed at the same time. It is difficult to expect a patient to be successful in creating these changes without dissociation. In such situations, direct suggestions seem to be more powerful than indirect suggestions. This has been recently confirmed by Lynn (1997).

The next important issue is to help patients to change a negative belief system into a positive one. Critically ill or injured patients often expect the worst. One good way to counteract this is to use a future-oriented technique, (Rossi & Cheek, 1988). Talking to patients about all the interesting things they will do once again, when they are all well, will accomplish this. To encourage them to visualize and experience this will reinforce it. Excellent results, using this avenue, have been accomplished and it takes no additional time. Furthermore, a positive view of the future in itself appears to be ego strengthening and integrating (Frederick & Phillips, 1992). Silence on our part is potentially threatening to the patient and even more anxiety provoking. Rossi and Cheek (1988) point out that it is important for us to help patients access healing sources within their own bodies.

Among the many conditions we see in the emergency unit, the use of hypnosis with burn patients is of great importance. Early treatment of burns with hypnosis, soon after an accident happens, often prevents progression of a first degree burn to second degree, or second to third degree. The suggestions should be directed toward antiinflammation, such as "keep the involved areas cool and comfortable." There are two parts to a burn injury. The first is the actual insult, the heat injury, and the second is the tissue's response to the stimulus. It is this tissue reaction which can be influenced with hypnosis. When the patient responds to appropriate hypnotic suggestions, there is usually no swelling, no edema or inflammatory reaction and therefore much less fluid loss. The rate of infections is also diminished, (Ewin 1992b). Chapman, Goodell, and Wolff (1959) showed that hypnotically-induced analgesia blocked the production of the peptide bradykinin. Ewin (1984, 1986a, 1986b, 1992b) published extensively on this subject, talking about his experiences in the use of hypnosis with burn patients. During many years of adding hypnosis to the routine care of burn patients, in addition to the administration of narcotics, he showed remarkable results. Though lacking controlled studies, Ewin's work has great value in documenting great success with "before and after" photographs of burn patients, as well as with videotapes of hypnosis for patients with burns (personal communication and teaching during workshops). He requests from his patients that they follow all his suggestions, to leave the treatment to him, and then sends them to their "laughing place," which is a typical dissociation technique. Patients with burn injuries have been found to be even more receptive to hypnosis than the general population (Patterson, Adcock, & Bombardier, 1997). This may be due to greater motivation, regression, dissociation, and possibly expectation, because of the excruciating pain, which they suffer during the treatment, which includes immersion in tanks for wound cleansing, and during dressing changes. Hypnosis is one of the most successful and appropriate interventions for burn injuries, and while it does not replace narcotics, it often dramatically increases the success of routine treatments through modulation of pain and anxiety.

Patterson, Everett, Burns, and Marvin (1992), in a well-controlled study, reported that hypnotized patients showed superior pain relief compared to a no-treatment control group. They used standardized hypnotic techniques in order to produce controlled, replicable effects. Since the personalized nature of hypnotic treatment is an essential ingredient, it is probable that their results would have been even more dramatic if hypnotic techniques were tailored to each patient's needs and preferences instead of using the same technique for every patient as part of a research protocol. The bio-psycho-social resources of each patient must be assessed individually in order to fashion a successful modus operandi. Erickson (1980) also stated that it is essential to evaluate patients' coping strategies and to recognize their need to be in control. In addition, he found the ability to experience vivid imagery and to dissociate is important. Patients needs are very different when they are vigilant and confronting, as opposed to when they are avoidant. Techniques must vary accordingly. With a vigilant patient, more detail and more involvement are indicated and useful. In comparison, avoidant patients do better with help in becoming relaxed, going inward, dissociating and experiencing pleasant sensations. When patients with high levels of pain use hypnosis, they show good analgesic results. This can be attributed to motivation, dissociation, and regression.

Appropriate hypnotic suggestions should be used to combat the guilt or anger which is present in most patients. Knowing that hypnosis can change perception, memory, and mood, reframing can be used for these as well as for the treatment of depression, which is so prevalent in severely burned patients. Helping patients to reinterpret their perception of the experience will assist them in changing their cognition and in turn help to diminish the affective part of the pain experience (Price, 1988).

Unfortunately there are very few places where hypnosis is used as an adjunctive treatment for burn patients. Patterson, Questad, and Boltwood (1987) state that it is interesting that a treatment technique that is so often held in question appears to be so effective with burn pain. This statement, even though it was made more than ten years ago, holds true today. Hypnosis is still underused in many fields of medicine, especially in the preparation of patients for surgery, anxiety provoking and/or painful procedures, and in the treatment of pain of various origins, such as burns. "Hypnosis should be regarded as a useful adjunct, particularly for patients who are having a poor response to standard regimens" (Patterson et al., 1997, p. 390). Hypnosis and hypnotic techniques should be made available to all patients.

As pointed out before, critically ill, injured, hemorrhaging, or severely burned patients are in a state of altered awareness, emotional regression with a shift to primary process thinking, and show dissociative symptoms as well as increased suggestibility. All of these characteristics facilitate the acceptance of suggestions and the effective use of hypnosis. However, in the emergency room, some of the patients may be very alert due to the increased levels of adrenaline circulating in their body as a result of the "fight or flight" reaction. With these patients, the use of a rapid induction procedure is advisable, which is authoritative and short. There is no doubt of who is in control. As a rule, these patients are motivated, in great need of guidance and, most of all, anxious to get relief of their pain. Barber's (1977) rapid induction analgesia illustrates this well.

An example of a rapid induction which has been very successful is Spiegel's eye-roll (Spiegel, 1972), followed by ". . . let your eyes close, take a deep breath in and as you exhale, let all your muscles relax, from the top of your head all the way down to the tip of your toes. In your mind's eye, I would like you to go to a very special place, where you were happy and had a lot of fun. It might be anywhere you can think of, and please tell me about it, where it is and what you are doing there." If there is no eye closure at this time, one could say, "it might be good for you to close your eyes, so you can better concentrate and really observe all the interesting things going on in your favorite place. In your mind's eye, you may want to play golf or tennis and you will notice that you are at peak performance. Or you might just go there with your eyes open, it's up to you." Usually patients follow this regression to a happy place willingly and rapidly.

Suggestions

Suggestions must be relevant to the patient and to the circumstances. Depending on where these patients go in their mind's eye, elaboration with appropriate suggestions is useful. Thus, one might suggest going to see a good movie: "After you buy your ticket, as you enter the room, you notice it is very dark and you move forward slowly to find a seat. After you sit down comfortably, you will find that there are many people passing by you and as you watch them finding their seats, you notice that you are getting more and more relaxed and more and more comfortable with everyone passing by you. Very soon the movie will begin and you will be completely absorbed by the action, paying attention only to the screen." With the suggestion that they will see themselves on the screen, involved in their favorite activity, enjoying seeing and feeling how well they are performing, how easy it is again to be in complete control, a very powerful spontaneous reframing may occur. Ego-strengthening is very important and usually successful in these situations. Future-oriented techniques, with appropriate suggestions, can do wonders, not only because of the distraction they provide, but also because they promote dissociation.

To a patient, who might want to be in a lovely, quiet room with some soft music playing, one might suggest, "As you approach a log cabin, in a remote, quiet area, you peek into the window and see that there is nobody there. As you open the door, you see a lovely room, with fresh flowers on a table. You can hear soft music and you even recognize the familiar tunes. You continue to explore the cottage carefully and because it is rather dark, you touch the walls to steady yourself, feeling the smooth wood, which has a distinct smell of pine. Eventually, you come upon a flight of stairs leading down. Being curious, you descend step by step and notice that with each step you take, you go deeper and deeper and deeper. (This helps to increase the depth of hypnosis.) At the end of the staircase, you find the door to your own, private room, where you are safe, comfortable, and where nothing can disturb you. Sit down on one of those comfortable reclining chairs and thoroughly enjoy just being there and knowing that you are safe and protected." Obviously one can elaborate on this, and make appropriate suggestions of therapeutic value at that time.

Some patients might want to go to a beach, where they can observe all the beauty there, again involving all five senses. If they went into the mountains skiing, they could enjoy the snow and the cold, icy cold, which can be transferred to a particular area and actually be experienced by the patient, especially in the area of a burn or an injury. It is always appropriate to congratulate patients on their success in following hypno-therapeutic instructions. Patients really do not know what is "the right way" to do it, how to follow suggestions, how to achieve certain goals and thus the need to be praised is very real. Praise will let them know that whatever they are doing makes them successful.

When in hypnosis, it is not necessary to be relaxed and motionless. In fact, one can be very active and involved in sports. Athletes, as well as people in entertainment and show business of all kinds, use self-hypnosis while actively involved in their performance all the time, intentionally or spontaneously. If one wants to portray King Lear effectively, one must imagine and really feel that one *is* King Lear.

For the development of analgesia, it is useful to suggest that a very powerful local anesthetic is being injected into the affected area, or if the area is extensive, a cool comfortable spray will be applied. The suggestion of making the injured area cold and comfortable is very important for limiting the vasodilatation and swelling which is a tissue reaction to the insult. To take the patient into the "control room" in their imagination is also very effective. "All your feelings are stored there, and with a rheostat you can turn *it* down and down and down and even all the way off." It is preferable not to use the word "Pain," as it predictably reminds the patient of the experience of pain, which might be quite powerful. However, the word "it" is neutral and may be interpreted in many different, positive ways.

When using progression, the suggestion is made that patients imagine sitting in front of a television screen, watching themselves playing basketball, or tennis, or whatever might be important to them. "Enjoy watching yourself being happy, skilled, and active in the future, when all is well again." Rossi and Cheek (1988) routinely suggest to their patients that they see themselves in the future, when they are completely free of their problems. Torem (1992) similarly has written elegantly on age-progression techniques which have been used very effectively, with many clients in helping to improve their athletic performance, be they athletes or people who play just for fun but want to improve their game.

Rapid, indirect induction takes but a few minutes and does not take any additional time. Cleansing, debridement of a wound, or X raying and setting a fractured leg can be performed as hypnosis takes place. Because patients are highly suggestible and in great need of help, they enter or spontaneously deepen hypnosis readily. It also has been observed that sometimes this rapid and indirect induction achieves deeper levels than formal, slower and more prolonged inductions. Scaba (1993) believes that this might possibly be due to greater responsiveness to this type of induction by people of low and medium hypnotic capacity, and most people belong into this category.

The same kind of rapid, indirect induction can be used in any situation where a patient might require a painful medical, or surgical procedure. Lang (1996) very successfully performed interventional radiological procedures with her patients, doing what she called "Self-Hypnotic Relaxation," clearly analogous if not the same as hypnotic techniques described here.

The emergency unit is just an example of one of many areas where, with the use of hypnosis, one can help patients to cope with situations which are frightening, anxiety provoking, and which seem to be beyond their control. The sometimes astonishing results are gratifying to the patient, the family, doctors, and nurses alike.

REFERENCES

Barber, J. (1977). Rapid induction analgesia: A clinical report. *American Journal of Clinical Hypnosis, 19:* 138–147.

Chapman, L.G., Goodell, H., & Wolff, H.G. (1959). Increased inflammatory reaction induced by central nervous system activity. *Transactions of the Association of American Physicians, 82,* 84–109.

Cheek, D.B. (1969). Communication with the critically ill. *American Journal of Clinical Hypnosis, 12*(2), 75–85.

Cheek, D.B. (1994). *Hypnosis: The application of ideomotor techniques.* Boston: Allyn & Bacon.

Crasilneck, H.B., & Hall, J.A. (1962). The use of hypnosis in unconscious patients. *International Journal of Clinical and Experimental Hypnosis, 10,* 141–144.

Erickson, M.H. (1980). Literalness: An experimental study. In E. Rossi (Ed.). *The collected papers of Milton H. Erickson on hypnosis* (Vol.3), Hypnotic investigation of psychodynamic processes. New York: Irvington.

Ewin, D.M. (1984). Hypnosis in surgery and anesthesia. In W.C. Wester & A.H. Smith (Eds.), *Clinical hypnosis-A multidisciplinary approach.* Philadelphia: JB Lippincott, pp. 210–235.

Ewin, D.M. (1986a). The effect of hypnosis and mental set on major surgery and burns. *Psychiatric Annals, 16*(2), 115–118.

Ewin, D.M. (1986b). Emergency room hypnosis for the burned patient. *American Journal of Clinical Hypnosis, 29*(2), 115–118.

Ewin, D.M. (1992b). The use of hypnosis in the treatment of burn patients. *Psychiatric Medicine, 10*(4), 79–87.

Frederick, C., & Phillips, M. (1992). The use of hypnotic age progression as interventions with acute psychosomatic conditions. *American Journal of Clinical Hypnosis, 35*(2) 89–98.

Kleinhaus, M., & Solomon, Z. (1995). Hypnotherapeutic approaches and outcome of combat stress reactions 18 years later. Part 1: Clinical description and treatment strategies. *Hypnosis International Monographs, 1,* 145–152.

Lang, E.V., Joyce, J.S., Spiegel, D., Hamilton, D., & Lee, K.K. (1996). Self-Hypnotic relaxation during interventional radiological procedures: Effects on pain perception and intravenous drug use. *The International Journal of Clinical and Experimental Hypnosis, 44*(2), 106–119.

Lynn, S.J. (1997). Hypnosis and memory: A workshop. 14th International Congress of Hypnosis. San Diego, CA.

Olness, K. (1997). Symposium: Pediatric uses of hypnosis: Mastcell activation in juvenile migraineurs who learn self-hypnosis. The 14th International Congress of Hypnosis, San Diego, CA.

Osler, Sir W. (1932). Third Edition. *Aequanimitas : With other addresses to medical students, nurses and pratitioners of medicine.* New York – Toronto: Blakiston.

Patterson, D.R., Adcock, R.J., & Bombardier, C.H. (1997). Factors predicting hypnotic analgesia in clinical burn pain. *International Journal of Clinical and Experimental Hypnosis, 45*(4), 377–395.

Patterson, D.R., Everett, J.J., Burns, G.L., & Marvin, J.A. (1992). Hypnosis for the treatment of burn pain. *Journal of Consulting and Clinical Psychology, 60*(5), 713–717.

Patterson, D.R., Questad, K.A., & Boltwood, M.D. (1987). Hypnotherapy as a treatment for pain in patients with burns. *Journal of Burn Care and Rehabilitation, 8*(3), 263–268.

Price, D.D. (1988). *Psychological and neural mechanisma of pain.* New York: Raven.

Rossi, E.L., & Cheek, D.B. (1988). *Mind-body therapy: Ideodynamic healing in hypnosis.* New York: W.W. Norton.

Scaba, S. (1993). The Phenomenology of the experiences and the depth of hypnosis: Comparison of direct and indirect induction techniques. *The International Journal of Clinical and Experimental Hypnosis, 41*(3), 225–233.

Smith, P., Barabasz, A., Barabasz, M., & Warner, D. (1995). Effects of hypnosis on the immune response: B-cells, T-cells, helper and suppressor cells. *American Journal of Clinical Hypnosis, 38:2*, 71–79.

Spiegel, H. (1972). An eye-roll test for hypnotizability. *American Journal of Clinical Hypnosis, 15*(1), 25–28.

Torem, M.S. (1992). "Back from the future": A powerful age-progression technique. *American Journal of Clinical Hypnosis, 35*(2), 81–98.

Chapter 8

HYPNOSIS FOR CHILDREN IN ANESTHESIOLOGY AND SURGERY

DANIEL P. KOHEN

INTRODUCTION

Hypnotic strategies and more formal hypnosis are very useful in pediatric anesthesiology and surgery to facilitate comfort and obviate and/or reduce anxiety during emergency room evaluation and procedures, preoperatively, in the course of induction of anesthesia, and postoperatively for comfort as well as cooperation. Hypnosis may also be used adjunctively for a variety of minor surgical procedures in the management of burns (Olness & Kohen, 1996), in preparation for and during dental procedures, and to facilitate comfort during injections or venipuncture for blood-drawing and/or venous access.

Hypnotic techniques and approaches with children and youth must be tailored not only to the specificity of their individual medical history and medical/surgical/anesthetic needs as determined by a thoughtful and thorough medical history, but also must be developed with an understanding of, and attention to, the developmental level, personal interests, and learning style and needs of an individual child (Olness & Kohen, 1996).

This begins with an implicit understanding by the clinician (anesthesiologist, surgeon) that children who are old enough to talk may well be able to give their own history, and that there is always distinct and unique value in speaking directly with the child. "Connecting" with every child is essential not only to understanding who they are and how they are experiencing their medical/surgical problem and their anticipation of the procedure soon to occur but also essential to the development of rapport which in turn will allow for the evolution of an appropriate, reasonable, and more likely successful hypnotherapeutic intervention. By contrast, speaking only or mostly with parents and cursorily with the child/patient may be problematic as it by definition may prevent one from ascertaining the specific needs of the child and, therefore, prevent meeting those needs, hypnotically or otherwise.

However, from a developmental perspective, it is noted that young children, i.e., preschool age and younger, may benefit the most from hypnosis by having the most important figures in their lives, i.e., their parents, act as their coaches/guides in rehearsing and conducting hypnotherapeutic strategies. In such circumstances, the clinician is challenged to understand the child both through personal contact and observation, and through the eyes of the parents who may then be shown and taught techniques to be utilized with their children before, during and/or after anesthetic and/or surgical procedures.

Being able to successfully utilize hypnosis with children–including and perhaps especially with younger children–is based at least in part upon our *belief* in the ability of children to tell us what they need and our ability and willingness to respond accordingly. This requires an understanding of who children are, how they think or don't know how to think at various ages / levels of development, and appreciation for the normal, and even predictable regression that often accompanies the at least potentially traumatic experiences of illness, accidents, hospitalization, and/or surgical procedures (Brunnquell & Kohen, 1991). While a review of child development in this regard is beyond the scope of this chapter, an understanding of "different approaches for children of different levels of development" is critical to effective use of hypnosis with children, and reference to developmental considerations is included in various of the case vignettes which follow (Olness & Kohen, 1996; Kuttner, 1996; Brunnquell & Kohen, 1991).

IN CONJUNCTION WITH CHEMICAL ANESTHESIA

General Observations–Children's Needs

For the child who is going to have a general anesthetic for even the simplest and quickest of procedures, an explanation of the details and purpose of the process in child-friendly and developmentally appropriate language may be the most appropriate and important strategy the clinician can offer in order to obviate the fear of the unknown predictably present in children. Such fears may be amplified by prior negative experiences with anesthesia, surgery, or medically-related procedures. Since it is well known that patients with a high degree of fear in anticipation of surgery require larger amounts of chemical anesthesia, it serves both the patient and clinician well when the clinician is certain to ask about prior positive or negative experiences with doctors, hospitals, and procedures in order to know what to say and how to say it that will make the forthcoming procedure *different,* and, therefore, better, tolerable, and maybe even a positive experience.

Many children's hospitals have for years offered preoperative tours for children for elective surgical procedures. Beyond clinical observations that such preparation is valuable for children (and their parents), several studies have found that children having elective surgery benefit from some form of preoperative preparation (Melmand & Seibel, 1975; Peterson & Shigitomi, 1982; Wolfer & Visintainer, 1975). Scheduled tours of preoperative and postoperative areas as well as of the operating rooms and the laboratory go a long way toward demystification of the forthcoming anesthetic and surgical experience. Concrete information about what will occur where, when, why, and with whom is important for anyone about to have a procedure, but especially so for children. In the context of such tours, children have the opportunity to see, feel, touch, wear surgical gowns, masks, caps, and to experientially sample the environment. These role-playing experiences effectively represent play therapy, are in their own right hypnotic, and reflect a kind of "future programming" or post-hypnotic suggestion that can and should help to prepare children for procedures. Therefore, of the many key questions by the anesthesiologist or surgeon preoperatively should be "Did you have a preoperative tour?" "What was the best part?" "Was there any part you didn't understand?" "What do you want to know?" Analogously, the anesthesiologist and/or surgeon should assure that the child-patient knows what the procedure is going to be and should be shown both on models and on their own bodies what will occur and what they can expect. While these may seem self-evident, often these tasks are relegated to those conducting the preoperative tours, and surgeons and anesthesiologists miss important opportunities for reinforcement of these [hypnotic] learning experiences if they do not also honor their significance by discussing them. A recent issue of *Pediatric Annals,* a journal of continuing pediatric education, focused on anesthesia and pain control (Tobias, 1997). In six separate articles, a total of one paragraph was identified which focused on the value of preadmission tour and noted "psychological preparation of the child and parents is extremely important to help families set expectations for anesthetic care and the surgical experience" (Rasmussen, 1997, p. 456).

In so doing, we are reminded to be careful not to allow our sense of honesty interfere with our awareness of the power of our words hypnotically particularly to children who find themselves in these spontaneous hypnotic states of increased suggestibility. Thus, we should avoid saying "this is going to hurt" or "here comes a poke." Instead, we must remember that since pain is a perception—nothing more and nothing less—we really cannot predict with any certainty whatsoever what the nature of a given child's (or adult's, for that matter) "pain experience" will be. If a child asks, "Is it going to hurt?" just as it is a lie to say "No . . ." so it is to say "Yes" or "a little." More honest would be something speculative that answers the question by empowering the child to alter their own perception in order to create comfort. Options, therefore, might include something like "I'm not sure how much it will *bother* you . . . but as you practice learning about turning your pain switches off and on, up and down, you'll be able to control any discomfort so it doesn't have to bother very much at all. . . . You'll probably be happily surprised to find how it doesn't bother as much as you wondered it might. . . ." None of this is deceptive, none is dishonest, and its intent, of course, is to empower, reframe, and create the opportunity for the perception of comfort. (Olness & Kohen, 1996, Kuttner, 1996).

Preparation of the Patient—The Importance of Rapport

General hypnotherapeutic suggestions for children may focus on comfort, prompt and expectant return of normal body functions, rapid healing, and a return to usual, everyday life activities. The latter is especially important since it is quite common for many children to be afraid of dying as a result either of anesthesia or surgery. Hypnotic imagery regarding a positive immediate and long-term future are, therefore, important. Examples are found in the case vignettes which follow:

Case Example: JoAnn

> JoAnn was a preschool-aged child when she was first seen in the Behavioral Pediatrics Program. Born with sacral agenesis, her legs "did not work" and as a young child, they were amputated so that the bones could be harvested in a bone bank for later periodic use in reconstructive spine surgery. Preparatory to one of her last surgeries about age 13 years, JoAnn asked for help with hypnosis for the surgery. She knew hypnosis for pain control, but hadn't used it in quite a while. She wanted me to "tell the nurses not to give me any morphine or codeine 'cause it slows my gut down so much. . . . I don't want that 'cause I'm always so hungry after my operations and they won't let me eat cause my bowel sounds are so decreased." She asked that hypnotic suggestions for pain control, hunger, and return of normal gastrointestinal functions be given during hypnosis practice. She asked that she not be given morphine or codeine unless she requested it. She assured me, her parents, her surgeon, and the nursing staff that she would take care of any discomfort with hypnosis, and that they should just make sure that there was some food available for her to eat postoperatively. After two hypnosis rehearsal sessions a month apart (the second a week before surgery), she had an uneventful 5–6 hour spine-lengthening procedure. Only Acetaminophen was required postoperatively for discomfort, and she was very proud of eating supper 4 hours after surgery. (Olness & Kohen, 1996 p. 270)

In addition to the many clinical reports like those of JoAnn and others which follow, recent studies have demonstrated the efficacy of hypnosis in modulating the postoperative course of children. Recently, Lambert (1996) studied 52 children ages 7–19 years who were to undergo elective surgery, and who were matched for sex, age, and diagnosis and were randomly assigned to an experimental or control group. All children and families received the standard preoperative teaching and preparation for their hospital stay. Control group children received the same amount of extra time as experimental group children (30 minutes), discussing the surgery and topics related to the child's interests. Children in the experimental group were taught hypnosis as guided imagery during their preadmission visit one week prior to surgery. Hypnotic imagery included a rehearsal of the expected surgical experience, and suggestions for healing, for minimal pain, and for uncomplicated recovery. Each child was told to become as relaxed as she or he wanted, and that each could choose to imagine and feel what was pleasant. Choices were emphasized, and each child was encouraged with suggestions of positive outcomes, such as "You may be surprised at how quickly you get better, what fun things you will do after your operation, or how little pain you will feel . . ." (Lambert, 1996). Children learning and practicing hypnosis showed significantly lower postoperative pain ratings and shorter hospital stays than children in the control group. State anxiety was decreased in the hypnosis group and increased in the control group

Case Example: Billy

Billy was born with congenital scoliosis and multiple other congenital anomalies. By the time of our first visit he had already undergone multiple surgeries periodically to correct the deformity of his spine, as well as bilateral plication of his diaphragm, orchiopexy, bilateral inguinal herniorrhaphies. He also had a feeding gastrostomy which was used for the majority of his caloric intake. While he had the ability to eat, he was described as "needing coaxing" and eating only sweets. As he got older and became more aware of the procedures, he developed substantial, even predictable, anticipatory anxiety and a dramatic, phobic-like panic response with the very mention of a forthcoming surgical procedure. His parents characterized him as "fixated and terrified," and with good intention they responded to this by deciding to not inform him about procedures until the night before he would have to be hospitalized for his next surgery. However, now that Billy was 5-1/2 y.o., very bright, and very verbal, it was not as easy for his parents to keep this from him. When the father mentioned their concern to a friend, they were referred to our Behavioral Pediatrics Program for assistance with anticipatory anxiety. When the father called, he summarized the history quickly, and noted that the next surgery was scheduled for the following week, only 6 days from the time of the call, and he was hopeful that we could "do something to help with . . . his anticipation . . . his fear of bad smells associated with anesthesia and his fear of pain." We arranged to see Billy the following day, 5 days in advance of the surgery. Over the phone I asked the father to tell Billy in advance of the visit that he was scheduled for surgery for next week *and* that the following day they would be coming to meet a new doctor who had no shots, is funny, has a beard, and has some "very cool ideas to help the surgery not bother or worry him as much." This use of hypnotic-like, expectant language was purposeful, with the intent of beginning to form an alliance with the father, and also to begin to teach him the use of positively expectant language *in anticipation of the impact that parental attitudes, demeanor, and behavior always have upon the feelings and behavioral responses of their children.*

Billy presented as a somewhat small for age boy whose almost non-stop speech reflected his intense anxiety about both past and forthcoming surgery. Very engaging, he spoke openly about the prominent back brace he was wearing "for my curved spine." For the first 10 minutes, we talked about his favorite activities in order to develop rapport, and then asked him to describe his understanding of the reasons for prior and forthcoming surgery. He was clear that he had come to see me "for you to help me not be scared." Intense in his description of how awful his prior pain experiences were, Billy also described with a fervor his dislike and fear of the anesthesia mask and its "terrible yukky smell and taste!!" In an effort to show that they were trying to work with Billy on this, his father took a mask out of his briefcase to show me, but Billy found even this to be aversive, saying "get it away from me!"

At the outset I asked Billy if he liked "magic" and I showed him the "disappearing dime" magic trick. He was then given the dime as an "anchor" to help him remember me, this visit, to practice his self-hypnosis he was about to learn, and "because it will help you feel safe and relaxed." His father was asked to facilitate this via by getting Billy a "special container" in which to keep this " special dime." Billy was then asked if he wanted to learn something "really fun" and he agreed and closed his eyes upon request. He was asked to imagine doing something really fun and he immediately said he was pretending to be a pilot flying a plane all by himself and going to Florida. Multisensory imagery suggestions were offered to intensify the hypnotic experience (e.g., "You're the pilot, the boss of the plane [= ego-strengthening, metaphor for being in charge of the body] . . . just enjoy it . . . tell it which way to go, this and that . . . *hear* the hum of the engines, *see* the beautiful sky, *feel* the great feelings . . .), and then he was invited to " Now find the switch for your nose and smell . . . tell me when you see it what it looks like" and he reported with an excited smile, "It's pink, and round!" Then he was asked to "Turn on the smell switch . . . and smell some good smells" (and he reported "pineapple and strawberry!"); and then to "turn on the yukkey smell (of the mask) just for a moment or two . . . and then *turn it off.* . . . "

Before we had begun, Billy had told me that he wanted help with "nightmares" and had told me a story about a ghost he had in one nightmare. He was offered the suggestion during hypnosis "of course, there are switches for lots of things, switches for smells and tastes, switches to turn off hurts, switches for worries and scared feelings, and lots of others, everyone has their own switches different from other people." Later he told me "my nightmare switch is in my butt!"

Finally, before this first 15 minute session concluded, he was taught pain control with switches: "Now that you know about switches, I'll show you about those switches in your brain that turn off hurt ..with your eyes closed or open (note: young children under about 6 or 7 may not wish to close their eyes during hypnosis and this must be appreciated, sometimes expected, and used to positive advantage by the clinician). You know those nerves that feel sensations like touch, hurt, hot, cold, you know, well, they go up your hand and arm this way, and up to your neck and then to your brain and in your brain to a switch . . . everyone has different numbers and kinds of switches . . . take a look in your mind (this is a typical hypnotic induction strategy for young children who hear the believed-in-imagination quality of the instruction, and then *do it . . .) and see* what shape and color the switch is for your left hand." And he did, reported first that the left hand had a blue switch and the right a pink but then that both were blue. "Now, turn it down until it's off. And check the other one, and make sure it's on. Now, pinch the skin on the hand that you turned off. On a scale from 0–12 with 12 the worst and 0 no hurt at all, what numbered is it down to? And he reported "3". He was asked then to compare this to how the other hand felt when pinched when the switch was on. After he had noted with astonishment the significant difference, he smiled and nodded agreement when I asked "Isn't that cool what *you did?!* (The use of "you did" is a purposeful ego-enhancing compliment it was him *and* that he *did* it, i.e., past tense.) Post-hypnotic suggestions were given for use of the switches "for any hurt that might be bothering during or after the operation, of course, there's at least one switch for the back . . . (which would be the site of the planned surgery)."

At the end of the hypnotic experience, Billy was told, "Now, just picture yourself getting ready for that operation next week, see how comfortable and relaxed you are and just before that mask starts to get ready with the sleeping medicine, switch the taste and smell switches to pineapple popsicles . . . right . . . great . . . and you'll be able to switch *any* smell or *any* taste to anyone you like—like pineapple—whenever you need to . . . what a great thing to know . . . the more you practice it the better you'll get." After he realerted, we reviewed the suggestions in his usual state of alertness, and he agreed to practice it twice daily prior to surgery, and to teach the techniques to his mother when they got home.

His father became very engaged with this process as well and later reported being able to use these techniques effectively with Billy.

Six weeks later, 5 weeks after the surgery, Billy was eager to talk about the surgical experience. Reflecting his sense of mastery of the experience, he enjoyed reporting at once that "I was scared" and that "I chose bubble gum" meaning the flavor of "Lip Smackers" that was put on the anesthesia mask to facilitate his comfort. He spoke very positively of having used the "pain switch" postoperatively but also wondered aloud, "I don't know if I should remember the surgery because I don't want to feel bad," to which I responded by telling him "well, you could just turn off the unhappy memories part . . . " and he liked that idea.

As he matured, Billy learned additional age/development-specific techniques to help him cope with and manage his generalized anxiety which would typically worsen around the time of another surgical procedure. In addition, with one to three "review and application" visits each time, he was able to quickly adapt his self-hypnosis skills to manage various other problems he encountered over time, including, e.g., (1) primary nocturnal enuresis (bedwetting), (2) sleep onset anxiety, and (3) anger management.

DURING INDUCTION OF ANESTHESIA

Independent of formal hypnosis, the anesthesiologist/anesthetist/nurse should use the opportunity of the immediate preoperative, natural state of focused alertness to repeat and reinforce what positive expectations were offered during preanesthetic preparation. Thus, like the appropriate guidelines for a high quality [medical] lecture (i.e., where we tell the learners what we expect to teach and how we'll teach it, then we teach it, and then we discuss what we taught and how we taught it), so we should tell the patient what we'll do together, then do it, then tell him what we did. In this fashion, repetition, as with repetition of therapeutic suggestions during formal trance, serves to reinforce and anchor the positive suggestion and expectation. This also insures that when and as the procedure actually takes place, it won't be the first, but rather the second or third time the child is hearing about–and now experiencing–the sequence of events and behaviors.

Linked carefully to the preoperative preparation, the suggestions offered during induction of anesthesia, therefore, should be language and format the patient has heard before, e.g. ". . . In a few moments when you begin breathing, the special medicine for sleeping during the operation, it will be just like we discussed. You'll remember the operating room and all of the nurses and doctors there to help you, and you'll be able to notice how you turn off the switch to your arm so the IV can go in easily, just like we practiced it together. . . . that's right . . . so you can begin now to just drift in your mind off to your favorite place, and I'll be talking with you about everything, just like we planned. . . . "

When a child is admitted to the hospital for surgery, a clinician skilled in hypnosis usually has time to get to know the patient and hopefully to help coordinate attitudes and approaches of the family and various hospital staff involved in the case. It is indeed unfortunate when a clinician facile with hypnosis helps a child develop positive attitudes toward surgery only to be sabotaged by thoughtless, negative suggestions of someone else who may have had a previous unpleasant surgical experience. Because of such possibilities, it may be helpful to provide the patient with a safeguard against inadvertent negative language she or he may hear around in the operating room before and during the procedure. It is sometimes helpful to warn children of this possibility and to suggest, for example, that they can remember positive images even if someone else suggests something to the contrary. Preferably, of course, all members of the treatment team should focus on mastery, reinforcing the essential idea that the child can be an active participant in the treatment process.

Case Example: Hank

> 14 y.o. Hank has Crohn's disease and after 2 years of aggressive medical management was unsuccessful in reducing pain, bleeding, and weight loss, a decision was made to perform a colectomy, with a temporary ileostomy, followed in a staged fashion several weeks later by a reconnection procedure. Hank and I had met originally about a year before his surgery when he was referred for assistance with hypnosis to help with abdominal cramps, rectal discomfort, and anxiety associated with his illness. He learned hypnosis quickly and easily: As a young adolescent absorbed with concern about his body image, he enjoyed the use of multisensory (favorite place) imagery linked with relaxation and was very pleased to learn how calm he was able to get very quickly when he imagined his favorite place (a fantasized vacation) and did progressive relaxation from head to toe. In addition, he eagerly and proudly learned pain control with the "switches" technique, and was able to much more calmly and successfully navigate the self-administration of steroid enemas during times of active exacerbation of his illness with bloody diarrhea. To accomplish this, Hank was asked to watch a

video of himself in his mind (a dissociative technique) in which he practiced hypnosis to ready himself for the enema: "watch *that you* sitting in the bedroom, imagining something fun, going into your hypnosis, and relaxing down your body all the way from the tip of your head to the bottom of your feet . . . that's right . . . now watch how when you're ready you send the signal to that butt switch to turn the switch all the way down, or even off, *because* you know *when* (not "if") *it's off then you won't have to notice any feeling of hurt when you give yourself the enema*, that's right . . . now watch that Hank in your video go from his bedroom to the bathroom and watch how he gives himself the enema he needs to feel better, and how much more easily he does it when he uses his hypnosis this way. *After* you have watched that long enough and have learned what you wanted and needed to learn, let me know with a signal (e.g., a nod of his head). Great, now, before you come back to the hear and now, let yourself zoom the time ahead to the day of the surgery . . . and notice how calm you are because you have been preparing yourself. And you know now what you didn't used to know, all about how to help yourself be calm and how to help the surgery go well by the messages you give yourself in your mind like you've been doing. So, *now* that the surgery will be starting shortly, remind yourself to go somewhere in your imagination where you're comfortable and happy, and keep one portion of your mind attentive to what is going on here so you'll always be mindful of that so you can do your part to focus on healing and healthy responses of your body. Remind yourself that during the operation, you help the doctors help you by remaining rested, calm, and clear in sending healing cells and signals everywhere they are needed, by having just the right amount of bleeding in the right place at the right time, and by programming your systems to rest now so they can begin to function fully and correctly when the surgery nears conclusion and you begin to awaken in the recovery room. That's good . . . and I'll be talking with you throughout the procedure.

DURING SURGERY

As it has been described by Cheek and many others that patients can hear during anesthesia (Rossi & Cheek, 1988), it behooves the anesthesiologist, surgeon, and other members of the surgical team to pay careful attention to the content and flow of language utilized not only before and after, but also during surgical procedures. The clinician knowledgeable in hypnosis who is a part of the surgical team may be of immense help in this regard by not only providing timely and repetitive hypnotic suggestions, but also by being a model for the other members of the team. Suggestions during the surgical procedure itself might well include:

- Pacing and leading suggestions that inform the patient of the stage of the procedure at the moment, e.g., " The surgeon is now doing the _____ and he says it's going well, and ahead of schedule...."
- Suggestions for blood flow control: "And you can allow your blood vessels to bleed just the right amount to give a nice bath to the area being operated on, that's right...."
- Repetitive suggestions for ego-strengthening reassurance: "You probably already noticed how very relaxed you are and how you are helping the medication to work very well ... and you're being a great assistant...and in another part of your mind you can just stay in your imaginary trip somewhere ... just right for you....
- Toward the end of the procedure, the clinician's hypnotic suggestions should turn toward a focus upon preparing to become alert *when the time is right, very soon*; upon healing e.g., "be surprised how quickly you begin to heal by sending healing cells to the area of the surgery, and noticing how quickly your body accommodates to the changes," and upon return to normal regular functioning, e.g., and "as you begin to return to awareness you can give your bowels instructions to start to get moving because that's normal ... and when they do, then you'll be able to be hungry and have something good to eat soon after you're awake" and "remind your mind and body how well they'll work together for comfort ... you may notice some sensations of discomfort here and there that are normal, and you can pay attention to them for a moment or two each hour or so, and then you can *turn them off so they don't bother you until the next time you notice* ... and it's *good to notice the discomfort for a few seconds each 2–3 hours so you can notice how healing is progressing, and how much less the discomfort is getting*...."

DURING SURGERY AND ON THE WAY TO THE RECOVERY ROOM

When possible, a familiar face and voice should greet the young patient as they alert in the postanesthesia recovery area. This "anchor" of a familiar voice and face completes the picture, and continues to fulfill the set of positive expectations that were created as part of the initial preparation for surgery. However, whether the person is familiar or not is probably less important than their approach and sensitivity to the needs of the young person at this time. Not unlike the focused, narrowed attention of the induced hypnotic state or the negative hypnotic state of patients in states of acute pain and anxiety states, this immediate post-operative state is one in which the individual is working hard to focus and concentrate even while struggling against discomfort and disorientation. Accordingly, soothing, comforting and *familiar language content* are appropriate. The nurse or physician who has not met the child before this time should nonetheless be familiar with their needs through the inclusion of notes from the anesthesiologist or surgeon who provided hypnotherapeutic preparation before and during the surgical procedure. Such notes should contain examples of the kind of hypnotic suggestions useful for this child and some indication of their particular interests and preferred imagery.

More formally, in the recovery room and immediate postoperative period, the clinician should resume the prior hypnotic relationship and continue the themes of positive suggestions for healing begun before surgery. Added to this should be an increased emphasis on (1) ego-strengthening for pride in having helped the surgery to go well, e.g., "I know you are very proud of yourself and we are all very proud of how much you helped by being so cooperative and calm before and during the operation, it really helped everything to go very smoothly . . . " (2) a repetition of suggestions to the tissues for rapid healing and return to normal functioning, (3) ability to provide control of discomfort through the "switches" or other techniques. Time distortion suggestions are often very useful in the first several hours to days after surgery. For example, "You will probably be surprised how fast time goes by. You know how sometimes when you go to a party at 6 o'clock and you're having such a great time and then in a while your Mom says "time to go home . . . " and you say "time to go? I just got here!" and she says "No, it's 11 o'clock" and it sure didn't *seem like 5 hours, did it?* Well, that's the way it's going to be. . . . So, here's what will help with that discomfort in your _____. It's important for you to please really notice and pay attention to it so you can tell the nurses and doctors how well you are doing...that will help with the medicine and figuring out when to go home. So, every (2 or 3 or 4) hours, turn the switch on full to notice the discomfort for maybe 1/2 a minute or 1 whole minute, write it down on the scale from 0–12, then *turn it off until the next time you notice it again in (2 or 3 or 4 hours)*." Such suggestions not only give the patient the power to understand discomfort as "gray" (i.e., between 0 and 12) rather than black or white (there and severe vs. not there). Clinicians can only hope to understand and help a child in pain by promotion of this essential concept that pain is best understood as a perception and as very personal, and that if we wish to understand a child's pain, we must ask them. Nowadays, the fundamental principle of pediatric pain management is "the child's pain is real and the child is the ultimate authority on this pain" (Kuttner, 1996, p. xiii).

IN THE PICU (PEDIATRIC INTENSIVE CARE UNIT)

Like the Emergency Department, the Pediatric Intensive Care Unit has at least the consistent potential of evoking spontaneous trance behavior in patients, their families, and staff, by the very nature of the tension, uncertainty, and often "moment-to-moment" behavior of the environment and circumstances.

Case Example: Joe (Kohen, 1986)

> Joe was 12 y.o. when he developed a fever and "flu-like" symptoms of abdominal pain and vomiting. Well-meaning family members gave him aspirin which eroded his gastric mucosa, and he came to the emergency room vomiting blood. He was quickly transferred to the intensive care unit. Though an IV was begun, staff were unable to successfully insert a nasogastric tube to lavage his stomach. Each effort to do so resulted in more retching and gastrointestinal hemorrhage. Absorbed in staring at his IV dripping, he was terrified and in a spontaneous, albeit negative, trance. He responded quickly to an explanation of the diagnostic and treatment options, being assured that the blood running into him through the IV was necessary to replace what had been vomited. When he understood the *reason* for the nasogastric tube, he was willing and able to easily "turn off the switch for the nose and mouth so the tube can go in very easily and then you can begin to *get well*. . . ." The tube was inserted easily and subsequent attention was diverted from the sensation of the tube's presence by inviting him to "breathe in good feelings and breathe out bad feelings." He made an uneventful recovery. (Kohen, 1986)

Case Example: Sarah

Sarah traveled from her home 1200 miles away to have spine surgery at age 17 for a congenital problem now beginning to compromise her respiratory status. The surgery went extremely well and she seemed to be doing very well until the time came to prepare for extubation. She was terrified that she would not be able to breathe without the tube and the assistance of the ventilator though all clinical evidence was quite to the contrary and had been explained to her by the staff. Whenever the subject was broached, she became sad, frightened, and increasingly anxious, with additional ventilatory demands. This "negative cycle" seemed to be self-perpetuating. A consultation was requested to help Sarah specifically with anxiety to facilitate extubation.

Though this was communicated to me with a sense of relative urgency, there was indeed no emergency. While it was clear that Sarah should be extubated sooner than later, instead it was communicated that it must be "ASAP" (= as soon as possible), adding an unnecessary (and arbitrary if not false) sense of urgency to an already unhappy situation.

I focused on developing rapport with Sarah, coming to know her and allowing her to know me, and establishing a trusting relationship, long before moving into anything called relaxation/imagery or hypnosis. In talking with Sarah about expectations for success, I told her with confidence and comfort that I knew that her brain, lungs, and respiratory muscles knew exactly and precisely how to breathe and could be relied upon to do so now that she *no longer needed* the added help of the assisted ventilation. Appealing to her intellect, I reminded her that her brain and breathing apparatus had 17 years of experience of healthy, regular breathing to call upon, and that was good and important to remember as she prepared herself for the *ease* of breathing *after* extubation. Without any formal hypnotic induction or speaking of hypnosis, these positive expectancies were offered to her comfortably and confidently, and paced to her ability and readiness to hear them and internalize them for her own well-being. I told her clearly and directly that I knew she could do it, that I knew she was scared and that it was both normal and okay to be scared and that's why I was there to help her, and that I would be with her throughout the quick and easy procedure of extubation. Further, I told her directly "you're going to be surprised when you discover how very easy this turns out to have been. . . . " And she allowed me to teach her some imagery and relaxation to guide her self-hypnosis in preparing herself for the extubation.

And it was easy. After I had met with her 3 times over 2 days, she said she was ready, the endotracheal tube was removed easily, she coughed and breathed deeply and then easily, and then sighed with relief, and then cried, and then laughed. Sarah made annual trips to the hospital to see her orthopedic surgeon and we enjoyed seeing and talking with each other briefly during these visits.

As Sarah sought a career working with children with disabilities and began to work on her PhD, she began to correspond with me; and I asked her recollections about her hypnosis. In part, she wrote the following:

"... On to my thoughts concerning hypnotherapeutic strategies. It is impossible for me to say what particular experiences created the fact that I feel I have control over my body. I have incorporated hypnotherapeutic strategies into my everyday life. However, I don't know if being presented with hypnotherapeutic strategies influenced the fact that I feel I have control over my body (emotionally, physically), or if I had a predisposition towards a sense of control when you came along, you presented what already seemed natural to me. What if I had not already had that internal sense of control? I suppose I would have rejected your ideas. But, as I remember, you were the only person with whom I would talk . . . my recollections of the imagery experiences we did together in intensive care. I remember the "walking down the stairs to lower pain" imagery. However, I mostly remember feeling at peace because *you* were there. I think . . . the person teaching the child hypnotherapy is the key. I think that the only reason I even let you come see me was because of the peacefulness in your eyes. The "teacher" has to have something inside them that interests the child. Children are more perceptive than adults and they know if someone is not "for real." The "teacher" is more important to initial success than the actual hypnotherapy. If there is not something about the 'teacher' that convinces the child to try it, there won't be a chance for success. . . . Perhaps this is not a concern because people who are interested in hypnotherapy self select . . . perhaps someone who would even consider teaching a child hypnotherapy would automatically have that peace . . . I don't know."

Case Example: Ellen

Ellen was 16 y.o. and near death from pulmonary failure from her cystic fibrosis. As she became increasingly short of breath, she became increasingly anxious and I was asked to see her to determine if hypnosis could be of help to her. I learned from her family that they had just returned from a trip to Europe that had for all intents and purposes been Ellen's "last wish." She was very sad that the trip had to be cut short after 8 days because of increasing shortness of breath and hemoptysis. Though it had been Ellen's wish to have no artificial ventilation and be allowed to die peacefully, many hospital staff and some family members found this choice to be "wrong" from their perspective, and sought to reverse the decision.

When I met her, she was edematous from steroids, very short of breath, and I could barely see her face as it was surrounded by a cloud of humidified air in an oxygen hood over her head and neck. She turned to greet me when I sat by the side of the bed. I assured her that I understood her air hunger and she didn't need to talk much, just listen. She knew that I had been asked to come and help her with "relaxation" and she smiled. I told her that I was confident I could be of help. I told her I heard she had just been on a trip. Tears began to form, and she said "Europe, we had to come home. . . . " I asked "What was the best part of the trip?" Without hesitation she said "Switzerland" and I said, "Would you like to go back there . . . now?" She smiled, as though she knew exactly what I meant . . . and I said "I'll help you . . . just close your eyes and listen" I reminded her in an inquiring way:

"I really don't think there is a need for your mind to be here, is there? Your family and nurses are here with you and your body . . . your mind can be in Europe, right there in Switzerland, re-enjoying the fun just as though you are there because you are in your mind, and I know you won't mind using your mind to help yourself be safe and comfortable during these last moments . . . we're here and if we need you back here we'll tell you, in the meantime you be there and here together." She calmed, her tension seemed to "melt" as her body relaxed and breathing eased perceptibly, and she smiled and went to sleep."

Later that day I prepared a tape for Ellen, a somewhat longer version of what we had just done. Her family would not allow anyone to visit during the following and final 24 hours of Ellen's life, but the one nurse allowed in the room reported that Ellen was very calm and that the tape had been played a few times.

IN CONJUNCTION WITH REGIONAL ANESTHESIA

As noted throughout this chapter, the essence of success with hypnosis with young people lies in the early establishment of rapport in the context of obtaining a history and identifying and facilitating the young patient's understanding of their problem and forthcoming procedure. This allows the clinician to develop a hypnotherapeutic strategy more carefully tailored to the developmental level of the child, and to facilitate this with imagery that is consistent with each patient's favored activities and experiences. With these as a template, regional anesthesia seems both particularly easy and also fun for the young patient. Perhaps this is because techniques that work well with children are those which facilitate mastery and don't at all conform to old stereotypes or "cartoon portrayals" of the all-powerful hypnotist who casts a spell on someone, or of the "hypnotized" individual "walking with eyes closed, arms extended in a 'trance', and doing the every bidding of the 'hypnotist'."

The "switches" technique works very well in this regard as it can be easily and quickly taught to a child fully alert, eyes open (see case example: Billy, above). This strategy combines both the concept of glove anesthesia and dissociative suggestions, which are easily combined to facilitate distancing from and altered perception of discomfort in an eyes-open hypnotic state. For children, this may be particularly valuable as the ability to watch what is going on permits the evolution of cognitive mastery (i.e., "seeing is believing"!) in addition to having "turned off" the affected part. The following vignette illustrates the value of this approach:

Case Example: Marty

> Marty, 17 y.o., was hospitalized in an adolescent psychiatric unit for acting out and disruptive behavior disorder, including some minor altercations with the police and refusal to comply with parental / household rules. During his time in the hospital he was known as the equivalent of "class clown" and had trouble with controlling and modulating his behavior there, too. When he developed a painful ingrown toenail and associated infection, a surgical consultation resulted in a decision to excise the ingrown toenail and drain the infection. Marty was "hysterical" and demonstrative in his demand for a general anesthetic, "put me out, man, I can't stand the pain." Marty had learned self-hypnosis just a few weeks before when right after admission I was asked to meet with him to help him with his lingering, chronic nocturnal enuresis which had been "unresponsive" to every prior intervention offered. After his success in quickly becoming dry with self-hypnosis Marty was willing to at least listen to the possibility that hypnosis might be useful in allowing the ingrown toenail to be surgically managed without gen-

eral anesthesia.

Marty had a previous experience with successful dental anesthesia. Both in one preoperative rehearsal and then during preparation for the procedure he was asked to close his eyes (induction), revivify the experience of dental anesthesia (intensification and deepening) *after* the needle and "novocaine" were already in his system, and signal when he could feel his mouth and gums and jaw feeling totally numb. (Revivification of hypnoanesthesia is best focused upon an area of the body that is *not* scheduled to be the focus of a forthcoming procedure.) Moments later Marty signaled and was invited then to "transfer all the numb feeling from your jaw and face *now* to one or both of your hands . . . and fill up *that* hand (a dissociative suggestion, i.e., "that" hand becomes numb much faster than "your" hand) with numbness *just as though you were pulling on a glove full of novocaine because you are filling up that hand with the feeling* of novocaine from your jaw. . . . " (This is the beginning of utilization and therapeutic suggestions.) Great, now, when you're ready, let that hand rest down on the top of your thigh and let all of the numb feeling move out of your hand and wrist and fingers into that thigh and down your leg, all the way down until it *fills that foot and especially that big toe that needs it the most,* to be calm, comfortable while the surgeon, Dr. _____, fixes the problem and returns that toe to normal." He nodded when he was ready and that foot (not "his" foot) was ready to have *extra* anesthesia added trans-cutaneously and by injection; and the surgeon proceeded with the removal of the toenail with Marty's cooperation. His cooperation seemed to reflect his belief in the suggestion that his foot could feel "just as though it wasn't even attached to you." In addition to posthypnotic suggestions for calmness and postoperative comfort, Marty was also given the (ego-strengthening) suggestion that he could be very proud of how well he had helped himself, and could even brag to the staff and other patients on the ward about how he had done this with "mind over matter," not even requiring sedation or certainly not general anesthetic. These ego-strengthening suggestions for pride are valuable and appropriate for anyone, but particularly useful and matched to the needs of this insecure and frightened adolescent. (ref. Kohen, 1986 in Edelstien et al.)

IN THE EMERGENCY DEPARTMENT

While a clinician has little time to get to know a youngster who comes to the emergency room, rapport can nonetheless be developed quickly. While the circumstances may often preclude the opportunity to explain hypnosis and evaluate several induction methodologies, explaining may in fact not be as essential as "doing." As so much of what we advocate with children hypnotically is about forming a therapeutic relationship and the careful selection of language, in the emergency room, the use of hypnotic language, strategies, and techniques without any formal induction is more often the rule than the exception. Of course *because* of the emergency, children are usually highly motivated to respond to positive suggestions.

Whichever clinician first greets a child in an emergency room has the opportunity to set the tone for the entire ER experience by understanding the value of communicating positive expectations at the outset, and in turn conveying an understanding of the situation and its attendant feelings. Thus something that "calls it like it is," gently and honestly, may be very helpful: e.g., "It's kind of scary to come to the hospital and be in this new place and have that (not "your") injury. It will probably keep right on hurting *some*, until it *stops.*" When the clinician acknowledges the child's reality, there is an increased potential that they will believe further observations and will follow subsequent suggestions. When the clinician acknowledges (to him or herself) that in an emergency situation (acute injury, pain, anxiety), people are often in a spontaneous altered state; of awareness, analogous if not identical to a spontaneous hypnotic state; this allows the clinician to proceed to approach the child with hypnotically, offering at once acknowledgment of the reality, reassurances of comfort, and positive expectancy suggestions for improvement (Olness & Kohen, 1996).

Erickson (Haley, 1958) has pointed out the value of commenting on certain aspects of the child's reality in order to turn apparently negative behavior to advantage. For example, one can comment that a child's tears are beautiful or that loud yelling reveals very healthy lungs. (These, of course, act also as suggestions for distraction and dissociation.)

Though everyone, and especially children, needs reassurance, vague comments to "not worry" or that everything will be fine are of little value. Much more precise comments may go further in promoting hope that the current scary situation will indeed soon change: The doctor who says, "I wonder if it will stop bleeding in one minute or two or four?" not only suggests hope, but also arouses curiosity that modifies anxiety and enhances cooperation. This is compared to the ill-advised, negative remark: "We've got to try to stop this bleeding. Now lie still please!" (Olness & Kohen, 1996).

After gaining rapport, the physician must explain what is going to be done, and how and when it will happen to the child. While in the name of honesty one often hears phrases like "This will hurt . . . a lot . . . (or a little)," this is most often very problematic and, therefore, ill advised. As it is really impossible to predict the extent to which a given child will experience the sensory and suffering components of pain, it is foolish to make such a prediction. So-called honest "warnings" that something will hurt may indeed end up limiting a child's creativity by imposing negative expectations, when, in fact, children are quite good at self-modulation of discomfort, especially when taught and facilitated by someone who believes in their ability.

Andolsek and Novik (1980) described four children (two three-year olds and two four-year-olds) who successfully used hypnosis during suturing of laceration, removal of a subungual hematoma, or surgical treatment of a thumb abscess. In each case, the physician facilitated hypnosis by asking the child to focus on the vivid sensory details of a favored topic [of their choosing] of discussion. Similarly, Bierman (1989) quickly established rapport, and then suggested favorite activity imagery for distraction and trance as the essential ingredient in helping a seven-year-old boy with multiple abrasions after a bicycle accident, a twelve-year-old girl with a scalp laceration, and a nine-year old boy with asthma and needlephobia. Kohen (1986) described six children whom he had not met previously who were also able to quickly capitalize on innate imagery skills in order to navigate suturing of lacerations and management of acute episodes of asthma.

Distraction may be used along with cognitive mastery by asking the child to observe body parts not involved in the injury. Thus, if the injury involves the left knee, the physician might check the other knee and also ask, "How does *this* knee feel? " In any setting where acute pain and anxiety are the presenting symptoms, the clinician *must* appreciate the reality and commonness of the spontaneously occurring, albeit usually negative, trance in which the child (or adult) patient is focused, concentrating narrowly on the injured part, the site of the illness, the sight of the blood or the misshapen bone, and as such is highly suggestible. This is already hypnosis. No induction is needed. The challenge, rather, is to connect with the patient and help them shift the negative trance to a positive one. This, too, is relatively simple and gratifying (and can also be quick) if one follows the principles described above and attends to development of rapport and honors and understands where the child is developmentally.

The easiest child a clinician skilled in hypnosis can help is, in fact, the young person in an emergency room whom she or he has never met . . ., i.e., there is no patient who is more motivated to make a change. So, given "half a chance," each child *will* follow suggestions, and *will* get better, *because* they are motivated, and our carefully selected words *will* facilitate them taking care of and charge of themselves and their discomfort. So, one kind of phrase which facilitates the beginning of a hypnotherapeutic relationship with an acutely ill/injured child in the emergency room is "Would it be okay if the hurt doesn't bother you?" (Thompson, 1978). Such a phrase "works" *because* it captures attention by asking a question children are not usually asked. In a way, in a child's mind it works *because* it is a "stupid question." As such, it works because it captures attention. In our experience, children always attend to this question, thus diverting their attention however long or momentarily from their anxiety/their pain/their fear. They usually immediately say "Huh? Of *course*, it's okay if it doesn't bother me. . . . " It also works because it is a different way of talking. Instead of buying into the relentlessness and hopelessness that the child in acute pain predictably feels (i.e., the fear, which is an inevitable concomitant, is always that the pain will not abate and/or will get worse), this kind of phrase implies a *choice* in the experience by asking the question, thus getting their attention. It is also different by calling it *the hurt* rather than *your hurt*. Such a reference invites at least the possibility of some distancing or dissociation of the person from his or her painful experience. And, it is also different by reframing the perception of the discomfort from "the hurt" to a "bother." Is it possible that all of that can happen or begin to happen with the turn of one phrase? Yes! Once the clinician has the patient's attention, focus can then be directed to additional hypnotic strategies to provide comfort. These may include pain control through distraction and dissociation (e.g., "did you see those cartoons on the ceiling? Which is your favorite?" or "I know this arm has been injured, but how is the wrist? And the other arm? And your knee down here?" or "Where would you be if you weren't here? Just go there now in your mind . . . that's right . . .") or anxiety management through favorite place imagery and posthypnotic suggestion such as

"I'm not sure exactly how *short* a time it will take to fix the (laceration, broken bone, etc.), but I wonder where you will go after you *leave here soon*. . . ?" Such positive expectant suggestions serve not only to inform and provide "future programming" but also serve to help the child by instructing his or her closest allies, the parents, in helpful techniques through modeling.

Often concrete information offered with hypnotic intent during such spontaneous hypnotic states of acute, severe illness can serve as powerful hypnotic suggestions which allow change to take place. An example is reflected in Kohen's (1986) description of the use of hypnosis to facilitate pelvic examination in an adolescent with acute appendicitis. Following diagnosis, the patient was given the suggestion that since she now knew what was wrong (appendicitis) and what was necessary (an operation) in order to become fine, there was no reason for further discomfort, since "everything that can be done and should be done would now be done" (Thompson, 1978). Analogously, she was given the suggestion that further vomiting would serve no important value and that she could have some influence on their being a minimum of bleeding during the appendectomy. Indeed, though an unusually long period occurred between diagnosis and surgery (20 hours while awaiting designation that the patient was an "emancipated minor" at age 17 years), there was no further vomiting. She had minimal bleeding during surgery, a rapid recovery, and ate 6 hours after surgery. Multiple examples of how and why to talk to and with children during emergencies can be found in Brunnquell and Kohen (1991) and Kuttner (1996).

CONCLUSION

Children who are about to undergo surgical procedures are commonly frightened and, as discussed, already in a spontaneous, hypersuggestible [hypnotic] state of focused awareness, narrowly and negatively focused upon their injury, illness, pain, and/or site of impending surgery. As helping adults, it behooves parents and clinicians alike to be mindful of children's vulnerabilities at these times. Depending upon a vast array of variables of their life experiences up to that moment, and upon their particular stage of development, individual children may think and believe that they personally caused their (or others') problem and/or pain through their misdeed or thought and may worry in turn that the imminent anesthesia and surgery represent punishment or retribution of some kind. Moreover, such fears are likely to not be verbalized but rather internalized as "deserved" and/or expressed in some other symptom or negative behavior. Awareness of and attention to these and related considerations should allow helpers to think carefully about what we say and when and how we say it, and in turn avoid further psychological trauma to children with pain and anxiety who are exposed to the threat of anesthesia and surgery.

REFERENCES

Andolsek, K., & Novik, B. (1980). Procedures in family practice: Use of hypnosis with children. *The Journal of Family Practice, 10*:503–507.

Bierman, S.F. (1989). Hypnosis in the emergency department. *American Journal of Emergency Medicine, 7*:238–242.

Brunnquell, D., & Kohen, D. (1991). Emotions in emergencies: What we know, what we can do. *Children's Health Care (Journal of the Association for the Care of Children's Health), 20*:4, 240–247.

Haley, J. (1958). *Uncommon therapy–The psychiatric techniques of Milton Erickson.*

Kohen, D.P. (1986). Applications of relaxation/mental imagery (self-hypnosis) in pediatric emergencies. *International Journal of Clinical and Experimental Hypnosis, 34*:4, 283–294.

Kohen, D.P. (1986). Hypnosis with acting-out adolescents. In B. Zilbergeld, M.G. Edelstien, & D.L. Araoz (Eds.), *Hypnosis: questions and answers.* New York: W.W. Norton, pp 399–410.

Kuttner, L. (1996). *A child in pain–How to help, what to do.* Washington, DC: Hartley & Marks.

Kuttner, L. (1986). *No fears, no tears: Children with cancer coping with pain* (30 minute videotape & manual). Vancouver, Canada: Canadian Cancer Society.

Kuttner, L. (1988) Favourite stories: A hypnotic pain reduction technique for children in acute pain. *American Journal of Clinical Hypnosis, 30*:289–295.

Lambert, S.A. (1996). The effects of hypnosis/guided imagery on the postoperative course of children. *Journal of Developmental and Behavioral Pediatrics, 17*:5, 307–310.

Melmand, G., & Seibel, L.J. (1975). Reduction of anxiety in children facing hospitalization and surgery by use of filmed modeling. *Journal Consulting Clinical Psychology, 43*:511–521.

Olness, K., & Kohen, D.P. (1996). *Hypnosis and hypnotherapy with children*–(3rd ed.). New York: The Guilford Press.

Peterson, L., & Shigitomi, C. (1982). One-year follow-up of elective surgery child patients receiving preoperative preparation. *Journal Pediatric Psychology, 7*:43–48.

Rasmussen. (1997). The Preoperative Evaluation of the Pediatric Patient. *Pediatric Annals, 26*:8, 455–60.

Rossi, E.L., & Cheek, D.B. (1988). *Mind-body therapy: Methods of ideodynamic healing in hypnosis.* New York: W.W. Norton, pp. 113–148.

Thompson, K.F. (1978). Personal communication.

Tobias, J.D. (Ed.). (1997). Anesthesia and pain control. *Pediatric Annals*, August.

Wolfer, J.A., & Visintainer, M.A. (1975). Pediatric surgical patients' and parents' stress responses and adjustment. *Nurs Res, 24*:255.

Chapter Nine

HYPNOSIS IN OBSTETRICS AND GYNECOLOGY

Patrick McCarthy

HYPNOSIS IN OBSTETRICS

Giving birth can be perhaps the most momentous occasion in a woman's life. For some women, the experience of delivering a baby is the most truly wonderful and memorable event in an entire lifetime of memories. For some women, however, the process of childbirth can be experienced more as an ordeal that somehow has to be endured in order to have a baby. Learning how to use safe scientific and effective self-hypnosis techniques can make the experience of giving birth far more comfortable and enjoyable.

Previous Reviews

There have been several textbooks and reviews from the last couple of decades that have discussed a variety of methods of using hypnosis and self-hypnosis methods in labor: Beck and Hall (1978); Burrows (1978); Charles, Norr, Block, Meyering, and Meyers (1978); Davenport-Slack (1975); Erickson, Hershman, and Secter (1961); Fee and Reilly (1982); Hilgard and Hilgard (1994); Stone and Burrows (1980); Waxman (1989); Werner, Schauble, and Knudson (1982). In recent years, Oster (1994) has proposed an elegant six-session model for individual use, but this takes six hours to teach and this reduces its acceptability to pregnant women and therapists. More recently, a two-session individual approach has been reported in two case studies (Sauer & Oster, 1997).

Research Findings

Clinical research findings from the last decade or so clearly show the value of using hypnotic techniques in labor. One of the largest studies of obstetric hypnosis took place in Wales, Jenkins, and Pritchard (1993), and compared 126 primigravidas (first-time mothers) using hypnosis in labor with 300 age-matched controls who were not using hypnosis. This study also studied 136 secundigravidas (second-time mothers) with another 300 age-matched control patients. In this research, each of the hypnosis participants received six sessions of individual hypnosis. The end-points measured in the study were the analgesic requirements of the women in labor and the duration of the first and second stages of their labors. The primigravid women who learned hypnosis had a highly significant reduction in the duration of the first stage of labor. (The duration of the first stage of labor is defined as the time from the onset of labor till the end of cervical dilatation.) These primigravid women who used hypnosis spent, on average, almost three hours less time in the first stage of labor than the control group. They also had a reduction in the average duration of the second stage of labor but the difference was not as pronounced as for the first stage of labor. (The second stage of labor is the time from the point of full dilatation of the cervix till the delivery of the baby.) The women who were using hypnosis for the birth of their second child also had a significant reduction in the duration of their first stage of labor, but it was not as dramatic as the reduction obtained by the primigravidas. The secundigravidas had, on average, no significant difference in the duration of their second stage of labor. Both groups of women who were taught hypnosis had significantly less need for analgesics during their labor. It appeared from this study that a hypnotized primigravida had the same experience of labor in terms of duration and intensity of labor as a nonhypnotized secundigravida.

Another study, Brann, and Guzvica (1978), from general practice in England, recruited 96 women. They were offered the option of either learning hypnosis or attending antenatal relaxation classes during their pregnancy. Roughly half of the group chose the hypnosis training and the others opted for the relaxation classes. This study found that the first stage of labor was significantly reduced in the hypnosis group and that the reduction in labor length was more apparent in the primigravid women. The women who opted for hypnosis training also reported other benefits, namely greater satisfaction with the process of labor, a reduction in anxiety, and help with getting to sleep.

Perhaps the most significant study, an American study, Harmon, Hynan, and Tyre (1990), consisted of a six-session randomized study which used group hypnosis training. This study recruited 60 volunteer women who were each having their first babies. In this study, the women's hypnotizability was tested prior to a randomization process. This is the only reported study to have tested for hypnotizability. The 30 women who scored highest on the hypnotizability testing were termed high hypnotizables. The 30 women who scored lowest were referred to as the low hypnotizables. Each group of 30 was then randomly divided into a further two groups. Half of the women would have hypnotic inductions. The others would not. The 60 women were thus eventually divided into four groups of 15 women: high hypnotizables with hypnosis training, high hypnotizables without hypnosis training, low hypnotizables with hypnosis training, and low hypnotizables without hypnosis training. This study, unlike others which studied hypnosis volunteers against those who did not volunteer for hypnosis training, compared groups who had all volunteered to take part in the study of hypnosis. This made the controls more comparable and valid.

Half the women received a hypnotic induction at the beginning of each group session and the control women received relaxation and breathing exercises typically used in Wisconsin, USA. This study found that there was a significant reduction in perceived labor pain in both the hypnotized groups and also in the high hypnotizables in the control group who did not receive hypnosis. Although the numbers in each group were small, this study of primigravidas also showed far shorter first stages of labor, less use of medication during labor, and more spontaneous deliveries than for the control groups.

MMPI* scores were taken before and after the training, and the highly hypnotizable women who had hypnosis had lower MMPI scores after birth than the other three groups.

To prove increased ability to tolerate pain, this study measured ischemic pain task scores during the antenatal training. (A sphygmomanometer (blood pressure) cuff was inflated until the pressure occluded the arterial flow to the lower arm and then the cuff was left

---

*MMPI (Minnesota Multiphasic Personality Inventory).

on the arm until it caused pain.) The women who learned hypnosis coped better with pain than the nonhypnosis subjects did. During the course of the training, they were able to tolerate longer and longer periods of ischemia. Most of the pain threshold improvements occurred in the high hypnotizables. This finding is in keeping with the findings of Hilgard (1979), who found a significant correlation between hypnotizability and the ability to alter pain thresholds when using hypnosis.

Benefits of Obstetric Hypnosis

Hypnosis training for obstetrics has to be both effective and acceptable. Acceptability requires that the learning of the hypnosis not be too time consuming nor too difficult for either the woman or for the therapist. Effectiveness requires that the hypnosis training have definite benefits. The research mentioned above suggests that the minimum benefits that one should expect from any obstetric hypnosis training program should include

1. a significant reduction in the duration of the first stage of labor (especially for a primigravida)
2. less perception of pain during labor
3. greater satisfaction with childbirth

Over the last seven years, I have developed an individualized yet structured approach to teaching hypnosis for childbirth to pregnant women which is both effective and acceptable (McCarthy, 1998). This program, which will be described below in some detail, has already been taught to more than 600 New Zealand women individually. The program consists of five sessions of 30 minutes in the final few weeks of pregnancy.

Group Versus Individualized Therapy

The Harmon, Hynan, and Tyre (1990) research indicates that group hypnosis training can certainly produce good results, but in clinical practice, even better results are obtainable when the therapy is individualized. Group work is acceptable in research work to confirm the validity and usefulness of hypnosis in obstetrics, but individualized work is crucial if the hypnosis training is to also be a truly empowering experience for each woman.

The only factors that a group of pregnant women have in common with each other are that they are all female and that they are all pregnant. No one would claim that one type of dress would suit all of the pregnant women in the group. Nor would one hairstyle, one pair of shoes, or one pair of eye glasses suit each and every woman in the group, so why then should it be assumed that one standardized hypnotic approach would suit all pregnant women? When an individual becomes pregnant, she is a pregnant individual.

Some authors and practitioners of obstetric hypnosis research and training advocate group lessons, principally to save time or reduce costs. It could be argued that since the pregnant women are each going to experience approximately the same type of event in terms of giving birth, then they might as well have identical training. However, each particular woman brings her own unique background of expectations, culture, experience of giving birth, and apprehensions to the training. She also has her own degree of parity, her degree of hypnotizability, and her own level of motivation to the training. She is undeniably female and pregnant, but most of all, she is unique. Teaching her as a unique individual implies teaching her both uniquely and individually. Group therapy for obstetric hypnosis can be effective, but in group work, the tendency is that the method itself becomes paramount rather than the focus being on the talents and abilities of the individuals within the group.

Planning the Training Content of an Obstetric Hypnosis Program

Most clinicians with experience in using hypnosis for the treatment of anxiety or pain control with nonpregnant patients wholeheartedly endorse and support its use in childbirth. It may well seem self-evident that hypnosis ought to be helpful in labor, especially if the woman is particularly anxious. Hypnosis for labor is a bit like motherhood and apple pie, often considered by people who use hypnosis to be unquestionably a "good thing." Hypnosis, when used for relaxation during labor, will certainly reduce maternal anxiety, but for the hypnosis to be particularly effective, it is important that the clinician have some understanding of the process of both normal and abnormal labor. Simply being in hypnosis is not particularly therapeutic. Hypnosis is a means of communicating therapeutic and helpful comments. The specific content of an obstetric hypnosis training program is crucial to the overall effectiveness of the program.

There is not a specific set of words that can be used in hypnotic trance to wonderful effect with all pregnant women. The precise words used by the hypnotist are not absolutely crucial. It is more important to understand the fundamental principles required in order to be able to use hypnosis to good effect in childbirth. This requires the therapist to have a good knowledge of hypnosis, obstetrics, and psychology.

Guiding Principle

The guiding principle behind my approach to using hypnosis therapeutically is that of hypnotic phenomena utilization. This same strategic therapy principle applies in designing therapy for both pregnant and nonpregnant clients.

Initially, I considered how to construct an obstetric hypnosis training program by considering how one could inadvertently use some of the classical hypnotic phenomena to have a bad experience of childbirth. In my role as a family doctor delivering babies for many years, I often had the opportunity to listen to women who had a previous awful experience of giving birth. It was very interesting to listen to the precise language of such women:

"The contractions seemed to last for ever and I thought the labor would never come to an end."

"The contractions seemed to be tearing me apart."

"I felt so exhausted I just could not push any more."

"The contractions were awful."

"I felt helpless and despairing and not in control."

"At one point, I seemed to be floating out of my body and looking down from the ceiling at the doctor and nurses."

Symptomatic Trance

I began my quest to design an obstetric hypnosis program by asking hundreds of women whom I met in general practice to tell me about their memories of labor. You can forget many things in life. You can forget your first friend, your first school, your first lover, your first car. Not one woman ever forgot that she had given birth. Women who were now grandmothers, having given birth many decades earlier, could describe their experiences in the delivery room to me. Often their recollections of giving birth seemed amazingly sharp and detailed despite the passage of many years. Frequently, they could tell me the birth weights of each of their children to the exact ounce. They could tell me how long they were in labor and who was present during the birth. In short, it seemed that their memory of such a momentous and life-changing event as giving birth became permanently etched on their brains. As I later discovered, the memories, while very vivid, where not always very accurate if compared with written records made at the time.

I listened carefully to the language of women who had a bad experience of labor and particularly to those women whose experience of labor was so awful that they had vowed never again to become pregnant. These women were fascinating. Their descriptive language was often richly symbolic and laden with emotion. These interviews were often deeply moving and it was a privilege to gain an insight into the impact that an awful experience of labor can have on a woman. Many of the women's recollections of traumatic incidents during their labor stories had a very dissociative quality. The women also appeared, without exeption, to have moderate to high hypnotizability. Some of the women had enough symptoms to justify a diagnosis of post-traumatic stress disorder (PTSD). There is very little available literature on PTSD resulting from traumatic birth, but a review has been published recently (Reynolds, 1997). As I thought about these emotive and vivid labor recollections and the triad of high hypnotizability, dissociation proneness, and PTSD, I formed a hypothesis that highly hypnotizable women were perhaps inherently vulnerable during labor and that their vivid imaginations could perhaps convert a difficult but essentially physiological labor process into a pathological and enduring nightmare.

Highly hypnotizable women have hypnotic talent, but hypnotic talent, can be a double-edged sword. They can use their talent constructively to lessen their pain and reduce labor time, but they can also unwittingly use the very same talents of creative imagination to intensify their awareness, their experience, and their sense of suffering. This negative hypnotic process is what Yapko (1990) refers to as symptomatic trance.

Giving birth ought to be a momentous milestone, but for some women their indelible memory of giving birth became more like a millstone. This psychological millstone could weigh them down for a lifetime.

Let us consider the various hypnotic phenomena that could spontaneously be produced during labor and consider what would happen if such phenomena were inadvertently generated in a negative and harmful way. We could speculate about precisely how a highly imaginative and hypnotizable woman, who is not trained in how to use her hypnotic talents constructively, could accidentally use hypnotic phenomena symptomatically to create a truly awful labor experience. Firstly, it would be helpful for her to generate prelabor anxiety by developing selective *amnesia* for all helpful and constructive comments about labor and have the ability, *hyperamnesia,* to remember only the labor horror stories of other women in great detail. Then, particularly if her labor was difficult or slow, she could start to become apprehensive and begin to wonder if perhaps there was a problem. Her imagination and a sense of pessimism could then increase her symptomatic trance experience. She could *distort her perception of time* and feel that she had already been in labor for ages and that her contractions seemed excessively prolonged and that the resting phases between the contractions seemed shortened. Then she could focus her awareness acutely on every uterine contraction and interpret the sensations in the worst possible way. This would result in the opposite of *dissociation,* namely *association* or even *hyperassociation.* Mild tightenings of the womb could be interpreted as pain, thus resulting in the opposite of *analgesia,* namely *hyperanalgesia.* Her anxieties and concerns could be further amplified. She could look backwards and reflect on all the contractions she has had and all the hours she has already been in labor. She could despair that the labor will never end and imagine that there is no hopeful light of expectancy at the end of the tunnel. She could start to imagine the baby becoming wedged in her pelvis and she could increasingly become more and more anxious, frightened, and tearful, with a growing sense of being "out of control." This would increase her adrenaline production and her nervous system would inevitably respond by tensing her muscles. The uterus is essentially a large collection of myometrial muscle. Tense muscles do not function well. Dilatation of the cervix will be slowed and impaired. Her progress in labor will further slow down. *Cataleptic* muscle rigidity in the myometrium could develop which would impair the dilatation of the cervix and slow down labor. *Mental images,* both visual and kinesthetic, could be created of the baby becoming stuck but the contractions continuing till something or someone tore apart. Barely controlled panic feelings would give rise to hyperventilation and increased catecholamine output from the adrenals, which would rapidly affect the biochemistry and further impair uterine muscle functioning. Feelings of helplessness could give rise to ineffectual pushing in the second stage of labor if despair set in or the pushing was painful. *Dissociation* could occur as a psychological defense mechanism and cause a feeling of detached unreality that was frightening and perhaps even perceived as a near death experience. Take away the last vestige of her personal dignity as with each push her anus empties her bowel motions onto the delivery table. Let her feel as though death would be a merciful release to make the labor stop and then allow her to realize that she won't die and it won't stop until it is over. From there, it's not too far to her developing PTSD and vowing never, ever, to be pregnant again.

The above might sound like a highly unlikely and extremely pessimistic scenario of childbirth that I've described. Unfortunately, my experience of 20 years as a doctor, and more than 2,000 births, tells me that elements of such a description are distressing not uncommon during childbirth, especially when the woman is both very imaginative and pessimistic.

Training Program

The program that I teach assumes that all of the above adverse phenomena are possible of being elicited in labor, especially with women who are highly hypnotizable. I further believe that after spending many hours in labor, perhaps always being in the same room or position, hypnotic capacity increases. I assumed that for each possible negative hypnotic phenomenon, it should be possible to teach the equal and opposite positive and constructive hypnotic phenomenon. In essence, I set out to create a hypnosis program that would prevent childbirth PTSD. The program, while personalized to each woman, aims to teach her specific techniques to recognize and generate the following hypnotic phenomena:

1. muscular relaxation
2. catalepsy
3. age progression
4. amnesia
5. anesthesia
6. dissociation
7. hallucinations

8. ideosensory responses
9. time distortion
10. posthypnotic suggestions

While it is true that virtually any woman can learn how to enter a hypnotic trance and that virtually any therapist can teach hypnosis, the key to a successful outcome is by working together as a team to establish the best teaching and learning methods for each individual pregnant woman. As a therapist, it is important to plan the hypnotic phenomena that we would like to elicit, but we also have to consider the talents and abilities of each woman and modify our approach. This will vary depending on her hypnotizability and her motivation.

When she has practiced and is capable of generating these phenomena at will, she will be able to readily alter her perception of reality and hopefully be able to have a better experience of childbirth. The program then consists of determining what order to teach and when to teach these skills.

Timing of the Sessions

Most textbooks recommend that one start obstetric hypnosis training early in pregnancy and spend lots of sessions with the woman trying to increase the depth of trance. This is, in fact, not necessary and does not produce the best results. I have found from considerable experience now that the best results are obtained not by starting the training early but by finishing the training as close to the actual delivery date as possible. Remember that the aim of the teaching is to enable the woman to be able to use self-hypnosis well during her labor. Like an athlete being prepared for a championship, you want her to be able to peak her hypnosis performance and produce her personal best when she is in labor.

The only problem, however, is that, unlike an athlete, she will not normally know the precise date on which her championship will be held. She does not know if it will be a daytime event, or an evening event, or both! She does not normally know in advance if she is to be entered in a sprint, a middle-distance race or perhaps even a marathon.

Preinduction Discussion

The first session is the preinduction discussion session. No formal hypnosis takes place. The preinduction discussion is best held about six to eight weeks prior to the expected delivery date, and I like to explain to the woman during this discussion that the proposed training will normally consist of four hypnosis lessons, once a week, each lasting approximately half an hour. I like to tape record each session and give the woman the tape to take home to use in daily practice. Many women have told me that they have found this to be very useful. Often they hear aspects they had forgotten and they can allow their partner and friends to hear the content.

Perhaps the most crucial part of any hypnosis treatment, or indeed of any therapy, is the initial preinduction discussion. I believe it is important to carefully listen to the woman and give her your undivided attention. Ask her about her expectations or anxieties about labor and her memories of any previous labors. Pay close attention to her words and her body language. Ask about her beliefs regarding hypnosis and gently correct any misconceptions. Specifically raise the issue of "control," if need be, and explain that she will always be "in control" of her mind when she is in hypnosis.

Do not make promises that you cannot keep. For instance, do not promise that she will have a pain-free labor. This will almost invariably lead to disappointment, as such a claim will seldom be true. Always underpromise, then attempt to overdeliver in your teaching.

During the preinduction session, assess her hypnotizability by asking her to imagine a variety of images which encompass various sensory modalities. This information will be useful in planning the therapy sessions. Give her as much positive feedback about her imaginative capacity as possible. Focus on what she can and has achieved.

I explain the benefits of finishing the program as close to the actual delivery as possible and then invite the woman to personally choose the date for her final teaching session and then we make the appointments for that date and for the three preceding weeks.

The therapeutic objectives of the preinduction discussion should be to:

  a. listen to her
  b. assess her
  c. be noticed to be listening to her
  d. inform her
  e. seed realistic expectancy and excitement
  f. have her leave the room keen to return to start learning hypnosis.

SESSION 1

The first hypnosis session is her introduction to hypnotic trance. This may well be her first experience of hypnosis and I have found that it is usually best to make this session simple, effective, soothing, and reassuring. I like to start with directed eye closure and to use very permissive empowering language. If the woman is initially tense, it is best to use a slow and gentle respectful type of induction. Use any simple induction method that will be easy for her to remember and repeat in self-hypnosis. I would normally then suggest that one use a simple basic progressive muscular relaxation, without muscle tensing, as a deepening technique (muscular relaxation). I normally start at the feet and slowly work through the muscle groups to the head.

When this is finished, explain that her current state of mind is what is known as a hypnotic trance and then ask her to verbalize what her trance feels like. Ask her, "What do you notice about the body now?" Note the presumption of change and the use of "now," implying that it is different from the start of the session. Using "the" body rather than "your" body promotes dissociation. You can ask her to explain what she notices about the body size, shape, weight, and temperature as a trance validation. Then gently ease her out of trance back to full awareness and ask her for further feedback on the experience. Then teach her a simple method of self-hypnosis. I usually use an index finger attraction method.

Index Finger Attraction Method of Self-Hypnosis

Ask her to hold her hands together in front of her chest, with the palms of the hands touching, as though praying. Then ask her to intertwine the fingers such that the tips of all the fingers rest against the back of the knuckles of the other hand. Then ask her to extend the index fingers till they are parallel, separating them by about 2–3 centimeters. Then ask her to use her conscious mind to focus on the gap between the fingers. Then state that if she is ready to go into hypnosis, the subconscious mind will choose to close the fingers spontaneously. Explain that when the fingers touch, then she is to simply close her eyes, then to take a deep breath in, and finally as she breathes out, to go back into a relaxing trance. When she does this, then ask her to focus on her outbreaths and allow them to take her deeper into trance. Then teach her a simple means of exiting trance such as counting to ten.

An audio-tape which includes this basic first session with progressive relaxation which is useful for almost all hypnosis therapy including instructions on the index finger attraction method of self-hypnosis is available (McCarthy, 1998).

Finish the session by asking her to practice what she has learned daily. Congratulate the woman on her hypnotic talent. Tell her that there is a difference between talent and ability, however. State as a truism that it takes technique and discipline to turn talent into ability. She has the talent. You will supply the technique and if she supplies the discipline of practice, then she will almost inevitably achieve her goal of proven hypnotic ability.

The therapeutic objectives of the first session should be to:
a. give her a pleasant experience of trance
b. reassure her about being fully in control when hypnotized
c. show her how to relax
d. teach her how to use self-hypnosis

SESSION 2

This is the main work session of the program. Ask the woman to put herself into a trance using the self-hypnosis method that she learned the previous week. This proves that you expect her to have practiced and allows her to show that she is in control of establishing trance. Then briefly deepen the trance and then commence constructing imagery of a beach scene with waves coming in to the shore. The waves crash and tumble on the beach and then they recede. Explain that she can use the sensations from her contractions to aid in the *visualization* of the type of wave. The incoming wave represents the rising contraction, the wave on the beach is the peak of the contraction, and the wave receding indicates the contraction fading. Invite her to feel a range of sensations. "Notice the breeze and the sunshine on your face." Waves have a sound and she can feel the crash and splash of the waves. The sea has a smell and if the spray touches her lips, she can even taste the saltiness (*ideosensory responses*). It is crucial to have the hypnotic imagery fit as closely as possible to the expected physiological inputs. Images of lying on an idyllic sun drenched beach in a state of total calmness are inappropriate during labor. Tell her that she can also forget the wave that has passed and thus develop *amnesia* for the associated contraction. She can look up the beach to the high-tide mark and see that the tide is coming in and that there is an inevitability to this process and that it cannot be slowed down or sped up in reality. Explain that she can use her imagination to choose to alter her perception of the duration of the contractions and of the resting phases (*time distortion*). The big contractions at the end of the first stage of labor, known as transition phase, are then *reframed* as surfing waves. There are only a few of these and they mean that it will soon be time to start pushing. "So you can take the chance, if you want, to get on your surfboard and ride those waves all the way up the beach" (*hallucinations*).

For second stage, pushing, the desired phenomena is increased muscle power or *catalepsy* which can be demonstrated by arm rigidity, and the best imagery that I have found that approximates to the physiology of the second stage of labor is that of squeezing a tube of toothpaste to empty it.

Age progression can be utilized by inviting her to imagine what it will be like in the near future to hold her baby in her arms just after the birth and be surrounded by happiness and excitement and also imagine how she would feel emotionally.

The final part of the second session is what I call *prenatal bonding*. I ask the woman to mentally communicate with the baby in her womb and to notice her baby's response. It is remarkable how frequently on doing this the baby suddenly gives a kick. I ask the woman to practice all these skills daily but especially the communication with the baby.

The therapeutic objectives of the second session should be to:
a. teach specific useful imagery for first and second stage of labor
b. teach amnesia
c. teach how to use time distortion
d. teach prenatal bonding

SESSION 3

The third hypnosis session is devoted to teaching two specific hypnotic skills. These are the skills of *anesthesia* and *dissociation*. A remarkably high proportion of the women I see can produce the phenomena of anesthesia and dissociation very easily. I explain how to use dissociation either partially, using "glove anesthesia" to produce an epidural-like effect and how to dissociate completely if there is an unexpected technical difficulty with the labor.

Dissociation Technique

Invite the woman, in trance, to imagine looking at herself in a full-length mirror. The reflection looks identical in terms of hair, eye color, and clothes. However, she will notice that the rings on her left hand are on the right hand of the woman in the mirror (or use some other unilateral feature). Then invite her to step into the mirror and change places so that she becomes the reflection and she looks out at herself. Then she imagines the concept of self sitting down and going into a trance while she, the dissociated, out-of-body reflection, comes out of the mirror and then floats off to a wonderful forest with an idyllic stream. Beyond the forest is a beach. It is the same beach discussed in the first hypnosis session. She can then experience the beach and the waves but now from a dissociated perspective. I teach her how to imaginatively observe her physical body from a distance in the hope that should she have a complicated or difficult labor that she will be able to spontaneously or deliberately choose to dissociate to a place of safety.

I then teach her how to come back into her body and become associated. I then teach her how to hyperassociate by asking her to place her hand gently on her thigh. I then ask her to notice her dress/trousers beneath the fingertips, then the feeling of skin, then the underlying muscles. I then ask her to imagine the feeling of the femur and even to imagine what the bone marrow within the femur feels like. At this point, the concept of hyperassociation makes complete sense to most people. I then explain that if she hyperassociates like that when having a contraction, she will be able to experience the full intensity of the contraction and more.

Glove Anesthesia

I then teach a glove anesthesia technique. The image used is of imagining a weird-colored glove. For some unknown reason, more than 60 percent of women spontaneously choose a purple glove! I then suggest that the glove has been soaked in a powerful local anesthetic solution. I soon speculate whether she has already noticed the changes in the hand yet. The suggestions used to intensify hypnoanalgesia and anesthesia are then a mixture of both direct and indirect suggestions using pacing and leading, metaphors, and lots of presuppositions. If this approach is very effective, then I give her the option of two suggestions: (a) either a pair of tights made of the same material as the anesthetic glove, or (b) that she step into a spa pool and an anesthetic liquid is poured in that is the same color as the anesthetic glove. Both these suggestions often produce lower body hypnoanalgesia. Women who have previously had an epidural for a previous birth can be asked to access at some level a memory of the prior epidural and use this to augment the hypnosis.

The therapeutic objectives of the third session should be to:
a. teach her how to dissociate or hyperassociate at will
b. teach her how to develop hypnoanalgesia in her hand and lower abdomen

FOURTH SESSION

I like the fourth and final hypnosis session to be as close to the actual onset of labor as possible, preferably within 24 hours of giving birth. It is best to use this session to clarify any specific details about the techniques. I tend not to teach any new techniques or hypnotic phenomena in this session. In this respect, I take my lead from good football coaches who like to lessen the pressure of training on their players just prior to the final game of the season.

This is the session where I particularly want to realistically praise her for her disciplined practice of the techniques that will hopefully permit her to show her hypnotic ability in labor. It is usually the last time that I will see her before she gives birth. I use a variety of simple yet specific *posthypnotic suggestions* during this session. One is about making a quick recovery from the physical effort of labor. Others are about the ease of breastfeeding and about making a smooth adjustment to the role of mother. Suggestions about sound sleep patterns and the ability to resume sleep if disturbed are also inserted. I encourage her to continue using trance after the birth for relaxation and specifically say that she can choose to be in a trance-like state when breastfeeding and feel a particularly strong emotional link with her baby.

The therapeutic objectives of the fourth session should be to:
a. ensure that the woman understands the techniques
b. give useful post-hypnotic suggestions for the post partum period
c. congratulate her and praise her dedication and commitment

Prevention of Postnatal Depression

About five years ago, I realized that I could not recollect any of the women who took part in this self-hypnosis program having developed postnatal depression. The usual incidence of PND within the first three to six months after childbirth is estimated at 10–15 percent. In the years since making that interesting clinical observation, I have specifically inquired about symptoms of postnatal depression. Wherever possible, I have asked women to complete the Edinburgh Post Natal Major Depressive Disorder Scale which is a useful tool for identifying the presence and severity of PND (Schaper et al., 1994; Cox et al., 1993). In the seven years that I have been teaching the program, to the best of my knowledge, there has been only one brief case of fairly mild PND. This occurred recently in a woman whose baby had a congenital jaw problem and was unable to breast-feed.

I would like to be able to say that this program truly decreases the incidence of PND, but these are only my anecdotal clinical observations and are not based on controlled prospective research. It is merely a hypothesis that this approach to obstetric hypnosis might be useful in decreasing the risk of PND. The women who choose to see me may well be from an unrepresentative group with lower risk in that often they are psychologically healthy at the start of the pregnancy and have good social support networks (Coble et al., 1994). The women are self selected. Prospective research is required and I would like to test the hypothesis to see if this is a true association or merely some extraordinary fluke. I would like to research with a group of women who have previously had PND and are pregnant for the second or third time and who are therefore at higher risk of developing recurrence of PND.

Many people think of PND as a very special type of depression which is caused by the dramatic changes in hormones which occur soon after the birth. If the cause were as simple as this, then the incidence would be a lot higher than 10–15 percent. Lots of researchers have studied a variety of hormones and have found no direct link between the incidence of and or severity of PND and hormone levels. PND has all the same associations and risk factors as major depression disorder in the nonpregnant.

Attitudes to do with autonomy, personal boundaries, demands on time, issues of control, pessimism, and a variety of psychosocial factors relating to the dramatic lifestyle changes that arise from motherhood are much more important than the obvious physical and hormonal changes in the postnatal period in determining if a woman is likely to develop PND.

Many readers will be aware of the writings of Martin Seligman, Michael Yapko, and Aaron Beck in relation to the treatment and prevention of major depression. Seligman's work on attributional style (Seligman, 1990) proposes that we respond to the triumphs and adversities of life by projecting meaning onto these events in terms of whether we perceive the issues as having personal, permanent, and pervasive aspects. He advocates that teaching people the specific techniques of optimistic thinking is protective against the development of depression. Let us examine the application of the above program against the criteria of attributional style analysis.

First, the personal dimension. I am at pains to point out to each woman that she brings her own degree of hypnotic talent to the training. She is the key factor. I am merely the technique tutor. She is the one who practices regular self-hypnosis. She supplies the discipline of regular practice. She deserves the credit for the success that she experiences antenatally. I give realistic praise for every achievement. Seligman calls this promoting *personal good.* If, however, she tells me that she has not found the time to practice her techniques or was unable to replicate a particular phenomenon, then I am quick to take the blame for the setback and I point out that this is probably my fault. I say that most likely I did not emphasize the importance of practice enough or perhaps gave her too much to do. Her lack of success is therefore almost entirely due to my failing, not hers. This is the attributional style called *impersonal bad.*

The next attributional dimension is permanency. When a woman obtains good results in practice, I tell her that she should be able to maintain these skills and do well in labor. I point out that obviously I cannot predict what her labor will be like, but I say that I know it will be better than it would have been had she not learned hypnosis. I point out that the benefits of learning hypnosis will be felt not only during childbirth but will be of great value in the weeks and months after the birth, especially if she continues to use regular self-hypnosis. This is called *permanent good.*

If the woman reports that despite practice, she has not achieved the results that she would like, then my role is to convert her belief from "not achieved" to "not yet achieved." I use a variety of truisms to point out, for instance, that it takes time to develop muscles and so it also takes time to develop hypnotic phenomena fully. I also explain that the reality of experiencing early labor is a great motivator to produce best results. A comment like "I suspect you are probably the sort of person who peaks her performance when it really matters!" This is an example of *impermanent for bad*.

In respect of pervasiveness, I tell the women having success in producing the hypnotic phenomena that they will be able to use these skills not merely in labor but also for lots of issues after the birth such as stress management, self-esteem, and confidence building. This is *pervasive good*. If a woman reports problems in learning a specific technical skill such as anesthesia or dissociation, for instance, I tell her that such skills are only a minor aspect of the program. I specifically point out what she can now do. At the very least, she can relax her muscles, she can concentrate, and she can remember what she has learned. I tell her that while she may not yet consciously realize how much she knows, it will be interesting for her to discover what unconscious skills she will be able to use during and after the birth. This is *nonpervasive bad*.

Michael Yapko's work with hypnosis in treating depression takes aspects of Seligman's work and expands on it (Yapko, 1992). He shows how to use hypnosis to reduce anxiety, increase expectancy, increase responsiveness, and decrease rumination. He advocates facilitating flexibility in distorted, rigid thinking patterns and espouses reframing meanings relating to faulty belief systems. Experiential learning is stressed. He also describes various aspects of depressive experience in terms of classical hypnotic phenomena. The skill-based approach of this program fits with Dr. Yapko's emphasis on utilizing specific hypnotic skills and on learning by doing (Yapko, 1997).

The obstetric hypnosis training program as outlined has the following characteristics:
1. time limited
2. structured
3. agenda
4. problem-oriented
5. ahistorical
6. learning model
7. homework
8. collaboration
9. active and directive
10. openness

These ten characteristics mentioned are taken from a list (Blackburn & Davidson, 1995) of the 12 main characteristics of the structure of cognitive therapy (Beck et al., 1979). The characteristics that are missing from the original list are the scientific method and the Socratic questioning style typical of cognitive therapy.

I suspect that this hypnosis program for use in pregnancy has intuitively incorporated elements of the important depression prevention work espoused by such experts as Seligman, Yapko, and Beck as well as incorporating certain aspects of sports psychology. This may explain why the incidence of PND is so low.

I would like to encourage the readers of this book (whom I assume will be largely composed of psychologists and physicians) to consider offering such structured hypnosis training for pregnant women and perhaps to conduct research into the prevention of PND.

Let me conclude by telling you what I frequently say to my psychologist colleagues in New Zealand about the use of obstetric hypnosis. It is a lot more easy and enjoyable to use hypnosis to treat ten very pregnant women who are a bit anxious than it is to use hypnosis to treat one very anxious woman who is a bit pregnant.

HYPNOSIS IN GYNECOLOGY

From Hysteria to Psychoneuroimmunology

When giving consideration to the role of hypnosis within the field of gynecology, we have to be careful about our choice of even the most basic words. If we use the words "Mind" and "Body" as representing separate and distinct concepts, we then immediately make a commonly-held, linguistic distinction that does not exist in reality. The notion of a mind-body complex as a unitary and indivisible whole is a fundamental and integral cornerstone of modern medicine and of clinical hypnosis in particular. Recent research findings from the discipline of psychoneuroimmunology (PNI) continually provides compelling evidence of the importance of psychological factors in causing a wide range of changes to physical tissue and of the equal importance of physical tissue changes on our thoughts, feelings, emotions, and responses. PNI is a fairly modern term that was only coined in the latter part of the twentieth century to describe the intricate linkage between the psyche, the nervous system, and the immune network.

The fundamental PNI premise of a profound and intrinsic psycho-organic connection is one, however, that has been intuitively known for thousands of years in the realm of gynecology.

The English word hysterectomy is used when referring to the surgical removal of the uterus. The word comes directly from the Latin word, *hystericus,* meaning of the womb, and the word *hystericus* itself comes from the earlier Greek word *husterikos,* this word apparently being derived from the long-standing belief that disorders of the womb were undoubtedly the source of hysteria, a condition allegedly limited, like the uterus, to women. No doubt it was some misogynistic man who deemed women to be inferior beings who initially proposed this particular choice of name for the uterus and thus began the long-standing belief. The Greek and Roman originators of these words did not have access to a DSM classification of the psychiatric condition that we call hysteria. They would have a layman's concept of the term. Interestingly, the lay definition of hysteria in my nonmedical dictionary (Collins, 1991) is that of "a mental disorder characterized by emotional outbursts, susceptibility to autosuggestion, and, often, symptoms such as paralysis that mimic the effects of physical disorders." Notice the use of the phrase "susceptibility to autosuggestion." If one substitutes the phrase "an altered state of mind" for "a mental disorder," then you have a definition for hysteria that is very similar and familiar to aspects of response that are associated with classical hypnotic phenomena. This particularly long-standing medical connection of the psyche to the soma is perhaps unique to gynecology. Despite the pejorative beginnings of this particular linguistic linkage, it now seems an undeniable truth that there are innumerable neurohumoral and other links to and from the psyche and the gynecological (and every other) organs.

Conscious/Subconscious Control and Influence Over Physiology

Some links from the psyche to the organs of the body are under obvious conscious control, whereas others are not usually under conscious control. However, these linkages are not clear-cut and distinct. For instance, we could consciously choose to control our hands in a very specific way, for example, to form a fist. We could also choose to lift or shake each and every finger of each hand individually. In order to play the piano, we learn how to move our fingers across the keyboard in specific and very deliberate ways. These finger movements of the novice pianist begin as quite conscious movements but with repetition, they become somewhat automatic (or subconscious). Similarly, learning the movements required when driving a car changes from initially conscious as a learner to subconscious. We can consciously and deliberately use our central nervous system to control a wide range of activities of the body. If we were asked, however, to deliberately, by sheer willpower, dilate our pupils, then we would have great difficulty. Similarly, we would have problems if we were asked to constrict our pupils or were requested to raise/lower our heartbeat at will. Asking us to increase or decrease insulin or glucagon production in the pancreas and liver or change capillary blood flow in our left big toe would cause bemusement and bewilderment. We simply would not know how to consciously will such things to happen. All of these physical changes can and do, however, occur in the body quite normally and naturally in response to signals that arrive not from the conscious but, at least in part, from the subconscious. This fundamental concept of the indivisibility of the psyche and the soma, and the influence of the subconscious mind on physiological processes is absolutely crucial to appreciating the current role and future potential of hypnosis and mind-body medicine.

In order to explain briefly the vital importance of this basic tenet to the use of clinical hypnosis in gynecology, let me firstly use by way of an example a nongynecological tissue such as the pupil of the eye, that is far more readily open to easy inspection of change. It is common knowledge that the pupils of our eyes can vary considerably in their diameter depending on the intensity of light in the local environment. If the light in a room gradually dims, then, without impinging on conscious awareness, the retina of the eye alerts the brain that with the background light diminishing, it is becoming more difficult to see clearly. The cones in the retinal fovea help us to distinguish colors and to work effectively they require a good supply of light. The brain receives incoming signals at a subconscious level about alterations in both color discrimination and light intensity and then sends outgoing signals to the muscles that control the diameter of the pupil. In response to these efferent signals, the pupils dilate to allow more light to enter. Similarly, if the light in a room increases, then the pupils will respond by constricting, using a method that utilizes the opposite mechanism. Interestingly, if the suggestion is made in hypnosis that the ambient room light has changed, then this causes the appropriate change in the pupil size in highly hypnotizable subjects despite no change in the light conditions in reality.

Pupil dilatation and constriction, however, are not purely a direct response to the ambient light supply. It's not that simple. There are several other factors that are important in influencing pupil size. If, for instance, we look at a person whom we find physically attractive, our pupils will soon dilate. This dilatation allows more light to enter the eye and so enables us to notice the person in more detail. Imagine being shown two almost identical photographs of the face of an attractive person, the only change being that in one photograph the pupils are digitally altered to appear a fraction larger. You are told that the pictures are of identical twins. If you are then asked to choose which of the twins is the more attractive, almost inevitably most people will choose the picture of the person with the slightly more dilated pupils. Even though the conscious mind has not actually registered the larger pupils, our subconscious mind picks up this subtle sign that may well indicate that the person finds you attractive to behold and has thus dilated their pupils. We tend, not unnaturally, to be attracted to people who seem to be attracted to us. This explains in part why many millions of dollars are spent annually on eye makeup which, in many cases, aims to achieve a similar effect on the beholder of the eyes, by making the eyes seem more noticeable.

However, it is also true that if we are fearful and worried, then our pupils will dilate, this time in order to allow us to see more clearly and to have more peripheral vision especially when we feel endangered. It could therefore be the case that the person who is looking at you, and has dilated pupils, actually finds you repulsive and scary.

There are a variety of other subtle, and not so subtle, means of verbal and nonverbal communication that enable you to make your judgement as to which possibility for pupil dilation in someone looking at you is most likely: sexual attraction, fear, or just poor light!

My belief, which underlies my whole approach to using hypnosis in gynecology, is that just like the pupils of the eyes, the breast, the uterus, the ovaries, the fallopian tubes, and even the actual eggs contained within the ovaries constantly receive truly vast amounts of information. This information arrives from both the internal and external environment all the time. Human beings have an amazing capacity to respond to such factors as attraction, fear, and a whole host of other influences throughout their entire body. Having received this constant flow of information via receptors located within the cell membranes of individual cells, this allows changes to take place at a cellular and molecular level due to expression or suppression of a variety of genes and gene products.

If you have any doubts that rapid or dramatic physical changes of a gynecological nature can take place in response to a significant alteration in incoming information, then the following quotation may well be of some interest.

In Jay Haley's excellent book, *Uncommon Therapy, The Psychiatric Techniques of Milton H. Erickson M.D.* Haley *(1973),* there is a quote by Erickson that I often choose to read to women with a variety of gynecological problems, especially infertility, while they are in trance, at about the third or fourth therapeutic session. I find it useful in the clinical setting to simply read the quotation verbatim without further explanation. This compels the listener to search for personal meaning as to why I have chosen to say these words and to deduce as to why I have chosen to read her the quotation and what she is expected to learn about the relevance of this quotation to her and her particular gynecological problem.

> . . . A man can have sexual relations with a woman, and it is a biologically local performance. The sperm cells are secreted, and once that process has been completed—the manufacture of the sperm cells—the man's body has no longer any use for them. They serve no purpose to him. They are useful only when the man gets rid of them by depositing them in the vagina. And so a man's sexual performance biologically is a purely local phenomenon and can be accomplished very quickly, in the space of seconds. It's just local, and once he has deposited the sperm cells he's all through with the sexual act. Biologically speaking, when a woman has intercourse, to complete that single act of intercourse biologically, she becomes pregnant. That lasts for nine months. She lactates; that lasts another six months. And then she has the problem of caring for the child, teaching it, feeding it, looking after it, and enabling it to grow up. And for a woman the single act of intercourse, in our culture, takes about eighteen years to complete. A man—eighteen seconds is all that is necessary. How is a woman's body built? Very few people stop to realize it—how completely a woman's body enters into the sexual relationship. When a woman starts having an active thoroughly well adjusted sexual life, the calcium of her skeleton changes. The calcium count increases. Her foot gets about a fourth of a size larger, her eyebrow ridges increase a little bit. The angle of

jaw shifts, the chin is a little bit heavier, the nose a trifle longer, there's likely to be a change in her hair, her breasts change in either size or consistency or both. The hips, mons Veneris, change in either size or consistency or both. The shape of the spine alters a bit. And so physiologically and physically the girl becomes different in as short a time as two weeks of ardent lovemaking. Because biologically her body has to be prepared to take care of another creature for nine long months inside, and then for months and years afterward with all her body behavior centering on her offspring. And with each child there's a tendency for a woman's feet to get larger, the angle of her jaw to change. Every pregnancy brings about these tremendous physical and physiological changes. A man doesn't grow more whiskers because he's having intercourse, his calcium count doesn't alter any, his feet don't enlarge. He doesn't change his center of gravity one bit. It is a local affair with him. But intercourse and pregnancy are a tremendous biological, physiological alteration for a woman. She has to enter it as a complete physical being... (Haley, 1973)

I often find that the detailed information of the physical changes described in the above quotation usually comes as a complete and stunning surprise to most women. Many people, however, having heard the above passage, comment, on reflection, that they have indeed noted at a subconscious level that sexually active women probably do look somewhat different but had never before given it any real conscious thought. Many young women who presented to me as their family doctor with some other health issue after commencing a sexual relationship have been absolutely astonished over the years when I spontaneously and quite correctly asked them at the end of the consultation if they also had any need for contraceptive advice. They and I had thought that I must be incredibly intuitive or even telepathic until I read the Erickson quote and understood that I probably must have been subconsciously detecting at least some of the subtle changes described above. The careful highlighting that Erickson makes of the multiple changes that occur throughout a woman's body in such a short space of time after commencing a healthy sex life speaks volumes about the capacity of the subconscious mind to produce widespread and significant changes. Hypnosis is also a means of utilizing the subconscious mind to produce widespread and significant changes. The message that clearly comes through from Erickson's words is that when a woman starts having regular intercourse then, at some level, her body realizes that with such frequent intercourse she is probably very likely to become pregnant soon. The changes are the changes in anticipation of pregnancy. These widespread changes occur quite subconsciously. She does not need to consciously wish to become pregnant. It does not matter if she is consciously aware or not of the likelihood of pregnancy; the changes will still take place. From this point, it is not too far a leap to the world of clinical hypnosis and fantasy where the therapist can rightfully say in Ericksonian style, "it does not matter if you are consciously aware or not of the likelihood of the changes that your subconscious can produce."

The explanation for these observable changes from regular intercourse is that there are a variety of neuro-hormonal and endocrine mechanisms that automatically start producing hormones such as calcitonin. These hormones change not just her pelvic skeleton but her entire body to make it more adapted and ready for the almost inevitable pregnancy that will ensue if she has frequent intercourse. The pituitary-ovarian axis and the predictable monthly changes in the ovarian production of hormones regulating the menstrual cycle, egg development, and endometrial change are well known. We also know a great deal about important monthly cyclical changes in pituitary hormones such as follicular stimulating hormone (FSH) and luteinizing hormone (LH) which affect the ovaries and uterus. Similarly, we know that the pituitary itself responds to a huge range of release and inhibitory messages from hypothalamic hormones. The hypothalamus and the limbic-hypothalamic tract are intimately connected to the thalamus. Increasingly, with the aid of advances in imaging technology, we are rapidly discovering that the limbic-hypothalamic tract is extremely active whenever we have feelings, and this area of the brain certainly seems to be associated with a wide range of emotional factors. This particular area of the brain also shows great activity when one is utilizing hypnosis (Rossi & Cheek, 1994). When asked, "Do you think this is all in my mind, doctor?" by someone who wonders if their condition may be "purely psychological," I sometimes might respond, "No, it's not all in your mind, but it might be in your limbic-hypothalamic tract!"

Thus the cycle of medical explanation turns full circle. As we enter the twenty-first century, instead of explaining physical gynecological changes as being the result of psychological processes such as hysteria, I now find myself explaining to women that psychological factors such as emotions, feelings, and consciousness arise as the result of physical changes within her neurons which are themselves determined by a variety of sensory inputs. These psychological/physical factors then impact on the rest of the body through the autonomic nervous system, immune network, and a host of other mechanisms, many of which are as yet undiscovered.

The phrase "limbic-hypothalamic tract" is my shorthand for a wide range of neural (and other) processes in other parts of the brain. These processes are not restricted to the limbic-hypothalamic tract. Certain emotional concepts, for instance, might be generated in the frontal lobes. Auditory associations, such as an internal critical voice, originating from the temporal lobes at the side of the hemisphere then influence these signals. The signals are further modified by kinesthetic or body-feeling messages from the base of the brain in the brain stem and cerebellum and altered by visual input being transmitted from the occipital cortex, which lies at the rear of the cerebrum. Thus front, side, base, and rear of the brain are involved in emotions and thoughts. The corpus callosum allows the left and right hemispheres to freely communicate. Left and right sides of the brain are simultaneously involved. Also what is happening now is influenced by our memories, both true, false, and distorted of what happened, or is perceived to have happened in the past and by our anticipation and expectations of what might happen in the future. Thus past, present, and future are involved in the genesis and construction of conscious and subconscious awareness. Try explaining all of that to someone in the first session when trying to establish rapport, and you'll see why it's easier to use a shorthand explanation.

Significant responses in the gynecological organs to psychological inputs as described above are not, however, limited to young women. Most women, for example, can achieve an orgasm during sexual intercourse or masturbation. However, there does not need to be direct physical clitoral or vaginal stimulation to produce an orgasm. Some women (I suspect they would be highly hypnotizable, though I have no evidence for this) can achieve an orgasm simply by being in the close presence of a lover or even by having the very thought of a lover or a sexual experience. This psychologically-induced orgasm can be just as intense as a physically induced one and the first time that it happens can be quite unexpected. The psyche that can produce such dramatic changes to the uterus as the rippling rhythmical myometrial muscle movements of an orgasm can surely affect not just the uterus but the whole body. A mother who is breast-feeding, for instance, will find that her breasts will fill with milk and start to leak from her nipples when she hears a baby crying

Eventually, I assume that our technology will be able to monitor and measure far more subtle alterations within the body. Until then, I take it for granted that physical, psychological, social, and spiritual influences directly and indirectly affect important aspects of gynecological physiology and pathology.

I stated earlier my belief that the uterus, the ovaries, the fallopian tubes, and even the actual eggs within the ovaries respond to such influences. Eyebrows might well rise at referring to psychological, social, and spiritual factors influencing the eggs. Some years ago, I attended a lecture given by Dr. Valerie Grant of Auckland School of Medicine entitled 'Maternal Factors Involved in Determining the Gender of Offspring.' I initially thought that this must be a misprint in the program. Every school child knows that the determination of the sex of the offspring has absolutely nothing whatsoever to do with the woman. Whether you conceive a boy or a girl depends purely and simply on whether the first sperm that enters the egg is carrying an X or carrying an Y chromosome. The eggs are formed even before the woman's birth. What possible maternal factors might there be? Dr. Grant has since written a fascinating book (Grant, 1998) that explores such issues and puts forward an interesting alternative explanation regarding sex determination. Briefly, let us consider what might happen if a woman, at some deep subconscious level, instinctively realized that she was better suited to rearing a male child rather than a female child. Is it possible that her subconscious could selectively decide to develop a particular egg from the more than 200,000 eggs contained within the ovaries that was intrinsically far more likely to be fertilized by a Y carrying sperm? This theory requires that the egg could determine by some means whether the sperm desiring to enter contained an X or an Y chromosome within its genetic material. The hypothesis may seem radical and controversial to those with no knowledge of hypnosis and the power of the mind. It may well explain, however, why a woman who has already given birth to four sons does not have anything like a 50/50 chance of having a girl in her next pregnancy. It may also explain why the male birthrate almost inevitably rises during wartime when women are under great pressure. The book is certain to challenge many long-held beliefs and is well worth reading. I suspect that it may initially be controversial, but, if true, such ideas may ultimately have the same impact as Charles Darwin's *Origin of the Species*!

As an offshoot of such an idea, consider the following. Women with bulimia nervosa tend to have above average hypnotizability on testing. Women with anorexia nervosa tend to have low hypnotizability scores. This latter finding in women with significant weight loss probably reflects not their innate premorbid hypnotizability but merely the consequence of their loss of brain mass resulting in rigid thinking. I suspect that anorexic women probably have above average hypnotizability in order to have the capacity to sustain the belief that they are overweight despite the obvious physical evidence of the reverse. Unfortunately, this negative autosuggestion of the need to lose weight can become locked in and the subsequent loss of brain tissue traps them in their delusion and robs them of the capacity to think differently until they hopefully eventually gain some weight and thus brain mass.

When a woman has severe anorexia, it would be disastrous for her if she became pregnant. The developing baby would parasitically have priority to take all the nutrients required for its own growth and leave her critically nutrient deficient. If her subconscious realized her peril, then to prevent her becoming pregnant, certain behavioral, attitudinal, and symptomatic self-defense changes would occur. First, her self-esteem would suffer. Women with low self-esteem tend to be less sexually active. If this failed to change her sexual activity, the next defense would be to reduce or even abolish her libido. This would further reduce her chances of having intercourse and possibly becoming pregnant. If all else failed, then the subconscious, as a last line of self-defense, would switch off her ovulation and menstruation. This would make it impossible for her to conceive. These changes, as described, are precisely what happen in worsening anorexia nervosa. They are called the signs and symptoms of anorexia, but they may in fact be the consequence of the subconscious successfully attempting to defend the woman from the risks of pregnancy.

Anorexia is relatively uncommon. Let's consider a more common gynecological problem. What would happen if an otherwise "normal" woman realized at some subconscious level that she was, at that particular time, unsuited to having a baby, perhaps because she was overstressed in some respect? Could she produce eggs that were unlikely to be properly fertilized? Could this be an explanation for unexplained infertility in the presence of apparently normal physiology in a woman with a very stressed lifestyle? Certainly the infertile women who come to see me are usually very emotionally stressed, but then I only tend to see them after they have been through the infertility investigation mill which can often be a stressful and impersonal experience for some. Does stress worsen infertility, or does infertility worsen stress? Probably both possibilities are true. While the precise mechanism of such inexplicable infertility is unclear, the obvious first step is to restore the woman's sense of holistic well-being as much as possible. This restoration of inner wellness can be achieved at a conscious level with counseling and logic or perhaps more powerfully achieved by working at the subconscious level by using hypnosis.

How I Use Hypnosis in Gynecology Preinduction Discussion

My approach to using hypnosis in gynecology is to work in a stepwise way from basic first principles. Each session, as with the obstetric program, is essentially based on teaching the woman how to recognize and utilize various hypnotic phenomena. Hypnosis can allow the subconscious to impact on physiology, pathology, consciousness, and awareness. We may never know precisely what particular words or hypnotic techniques to use to specifically elicit a particular desired response. Fortunately, it is not essential to know the words precisely. I do not work from a recipe book type approach to each individual gynecological condition. You will not find in this chapter specific spiels about pathology that are appropriate for all women presenting with common gynecological conditions such as dysmenorrhoea, polycystic ovarian disease, menorrhagia, or endometriosis. Just like the obstetric program, it is more important to teach the hypnotic skills that each woman can utilize in a way that is most appropriate for her. A standardized, disease-based approach could well be effective in a small number of cases, but the chances of being able to supply the correct words to significantly alter each individual woman's unique physiological and pathological gynecological processes in the desired way are remote. Such an approach would be akin to using a magical incantation. Effective and influential language, the basic tool of hypnosis, is, of course, important, but the principal goal of each therapeutic session and the goal of therapy must be clearly kept in mind. I believe that each session should be aimed at enhancing some important aspect of the woman's physical, psychological, social, or spiritual environment. My overall clinical goal is to successively provide a series of self-hypnosis tools that the client can utilize to help her attempt to reach her stated therapeutic goals. Each session should provide the client with at least one new tool. Hopefully, if the approach is being therapeutic, then the client will learn how best to use these psychological techniques so that her symptoms decrease in frequency and/or severity as she reaches and achieves her goals. The more self-hypnosis skills that a woman learns and masters then the more her self-esteem rises. As she uses self-hypnosis to feel more in control of her life, then she can usually cope better with her symptoms or at least not be so bothered by them.

The number and nature of the hypnosis skills that need to be learned to allow a feeling of control determine the overall length of therapy. Simple gynecological issues that are fairly clearly exacerbated by stress and anxiety may respond quite rapidly in fact to just a few sessions of learning some fairly basic self-hypnosis techniques which teach the woman how to be in control of her stress. Other problems commonly associated with gynecological pathology, such as pain, insomnia, or depression, require more specific techniques to address these issues adequately.

My way of working is not necessarily a better or more appropriate way for you to work. Your clinical culture and environment may be very different from mine. Please feel free to adapt my approach to suit your own circumstances. Briefly, I qualified as a doctor in 1980 and have a long background in family medicine and obstetrics. Since 1997, I have run a busy practice principally specializing in the medical use of hypnosis in Wellington, New Zealand. I am referred a wide range of medical and psychological problems. I treat about 40 to 50 people each week using hypnosis and would commonly see an average of four women presenting specifically with gynecological problems each week. These women are mostly referred by their gynecologist. A gynecologist is obviously the best-qualified person to perform whatever surgery and prescribe any hormonal therapy that is required to remove or alter diseased tissue. The gynecologists consider that my role as a medical hypnosis specialist is to augment and compliment at the psychological level the physical surgical and medical gynecological interventions they perform. I see my role as that of teaching self-hypnosis to empower women to make use of their own internal resources. The most common gynecological condition that I see is that of endometriosis, and certainly there seems to be a strong and seemingly common association between stress and problematic endometriosis. I do not say that stress is causative of endometriosis, but certainly the two conditions commonly coexist.

My consultation sessions are usually only 30 minutes long. I tape record every consultation and then give the tape to the woman to take away at the end of each session. Some women listen to the tapes over and over. Some are amazed at the content they have forgotten. Many women are reassured that I will not say anything outrageous when I know that it will all be tape-recorded and that I'm confident for her to take the tape away. In brief, I find that taping every moment of each and every consultation has proved very useful for a huge variety of reasons and I would wholeheartedly recommend this practice.

When a woman with a gynecological problem sees me for the first time with a view to the possibility of learning self-hypnosis, my initial consultation aim is not to seek a cure of her problem but principally to develop a sense of rapport and consider a reasonable plan of action. I prefer that patients be seen only with an initial letter of referral from their own family doctor, gynecologist, or midwife. People normally trust and respect their regular health provider and if that person is happy to refer them to me for consideration of hypnosis, then I almost inevitably gain some initial degree of reflected trust which is based on the personal recommendation of their regular clinician.

The first few seconds of the first consultation regarding the potential use of hypnosis are vital. The patient's initial impressions are crucially important to influence. I aim to project impressions of compassion, caring, interest, safety, and professional excellence. After a few initial courtesies, I ask the woman to explain in her own words why she has come. Often she may have come because she has a specific gynecological problem such as endometriosis, pelvic pain, unexplained infertility, or some sexual dysfunction such as vaginismus or dyspareunia. Many women with a variety of gynecological problems and symptoms come, not to directly address their specific pelvic problems, but instead to help them deal with symptoms such as anxiety, stress, depression, pain, insomnia, or other issues that often accompany their particular gynecological problems. Interestingly, despite hundreds of consultations, seldom has any woman with a gynecological complaint presented with formal psychiatric symptoms indicative of hysteria.

One concern worth raising that many women with gynecological problems often have is that I may want to use the history taking or the hypnosis sessions to explore her past in great detail in order to discover the so-called "cause" of her symptoms. She may be worried that I will want to ask her detailed questions about any possible history of sexual abuse or about her sexual experiences. While such issues may be relevant to her presenting complaint, I will often firmly state my personal belief that solutions to her problems firmly lie in the future. In order to find a solution, it is not essential and often not helpful to explore the past and open up old wounds (or even worse, inadvertently create false memories of old wounds based on inappropriate therapist beliefs as to causation). Michael Yapko explores and explains many of these issues well in a balanced and sensitive way (Yapko, 1994). My statement that I do not believe it is necessary to explore the past in any detail to provide her with help to reach her therapeutic goal is almost universally greeted with a huge sigh of relief. This is common in women who may have already spent ages in therapy going over and over the past. You can get a lot of vital information and develop a lot of rapport and trust by simply asking a nondirective follow-up question. " In brief terms, do you think that there is anything in your personal history that you think that I need or ought to know in order to help you?"

The fundamental principles of therapy that apply to hypnosis in any therapeutic session apply equally to gynecology. The first meeting, as stated above, should consist of history taking and seeding expectancy and hope. The former requires listening. It also requires proving that you have indeed carefully listened. The judicious use of verbatim feedback can be a useful way of proving that you are listening. In simple terms, you obviously have to have been listening to someone very carefully in order to repeat her words verbatim. Having taken a history of the presenting complaint, I find it useful to then ask the woman to outline her expectations of what therapy might achieve. The aim of this question is to ascertain if her expectations of hypnosis are reasonable and realistic. Most people that I meet do not have much experience of the clinical use of hypnosis and usually have very little or few expectations.

I then ask each woman to explain her goals of therapy. It is far better if her goals can be expressed in positive, definable, and preferably measurable terms. This is very difficult for many people to initially do especially if there is an element of depression. It is usually fairly easy to talk instead about what you do not want. You usually don't want your current pain, anxiety, etc. It is much harder, however, to state clearly what you do want. I prefer the goals of therapy to be defined as specifically as possible. I often say that I like to have a clear idea of what would define therapeutic success before we start therapy. A useful way to do this is to ask a double question: "If I had some sort of magic wand and you could somehow be well, what would you be like? Can you tell me what it would be like to no longer be so bothered by "your problem?" (Note how in the preceding two sentences the concepts of "well" and "no longer be so bothered" are interchangeable.) In order for the woman to answer these questions, she has to imagine a future scenario in which she is no longer bothered by her symptoms or problems. Now we are already in the world of "suppose." Officially, we have not started the "therapy" yet, but the seeding process has already begun. The aim of the seeding process is to facilitate her expectancy that there is at least the possibility that her situation might change. Seeding may well include explaining hypnosis and correcting any misconceptions about hypnosis. For further ideas on seeding see Jeff Zeig's ideas about seeding (Zeig, 1990) and about what he calls gift-wrapping therapy.

It is important to ensure, however, that you do not promise what you cannot deliver. There is a good rule of business and customer satisfaction that applies equally to therapy. If you overpromise and then underdeliver, then this will often cause customer dissatisfaction. Strive instead always to underpromise and then seek constantly to overdeliver. It is often good to formally confirm that you have accomplished this at the end of the first session by stating, "I don't believe that I've actually promised you anything at all. I don't and obviously cannot know how well you will do. I can promise, however, that we will work as a team to see what can be achieved by you learning how to use hypnosis."

First Hypnosis Session

Having used the first session for history taking and seeding expectancy the woman usually returns one week later. A small proportion of women report on the return visit that, to their surprise, they already feel more relaxed or significantly better in some way after the first session despite no formal therapy having taken place. Often, these women may have listened to the tape recording of the introductory session several times during the week. Listening to a tape recording of yourself outlining your history can have a rather dissociative quality. I often explain to such women that replaying the tape is rather like listening to a radio chat show in that it allows you to check if you totally agree with the "woman on the tape." Whether or not there has been any improvement, we then proceed to the first session of actual hypnosis. After initial courtesies, I usually invite the woman to close her eyes and then "simply listen to my voice as though you were listening to a play on the radio. All you have to do is imagine the scenery suggested by my words."

I firmly believe that the learning process of how to make the best use of self-hypnosis is very like the learning process of how to play a musical instrument, learning how to play a sport or learning how to perform a ballet dance. You have to start with the fundamental basics in all these disciplines and then build up from the basics. In one's first ballet class, for instance, every novice learns where her arms and legs precisely should be placed for the pose known as first position. She then learns the specifics of second position, third position, and so on. The role of the therapist using hypnosis is often that of a self-hypnosis technique tutor. This means that the therapist will repeat the same basic beginner lessons to hundreds and hundreds of people, endeavoring to ensure that there is the same enthusiasm and interest given to the thousandth pupil as given to the first. Each woman's first experience of hypnosis must be simple, safe, enjoyable, and able to produce some immediate demonstrable benefit such as relaxation at the very least. The woman should feel empowered by the experience and keen to learn more. You can easily judge your success by the percentage of paying customers eagerly returning for their next session. There is little to be gained by employing technically elegant hypnosis, from whatever latest fad or theoretical background, which feeds the ego of the therapist, if the client chooses not to return for further sessions!

For me, the hypnosis equivalent of teaching the basics of first and second ballet position is that I tend to teach the same initial induction and first and second hypnosis sessions to about 95 percent of my patients almost irrespective of their presenting problem. These first two sessions focus on the basic skills of relaxation and putting ones problems off to one side symbolically. Unless the person has current pain > 50 on a 0–100 scale, I tend to use in the first session a fairly standard conversational induction of external environment awareness followed by internal awareness. This induction then leads on to a simple metaphor with an indirect age regression suggestion to childhood memories, about using a magnifying glass to focus the sun's rays to set fire to paper. This metaphor indirectly conveys to the woman that I now want her to really concentrate her focus of attention. The induction then flows into a simple progressive muscle relaxation, with relatively minor but absolutely crucial personalized alterations to make the session appear very individualized to that woman. The progressive relaxation is thus used principally as a deepening technique. (Doing this form of deepening with someone in great pain merely invites her to focus on her pain and so ensures that in a single session you lose a client and discredit hypnosis.) I find it best to start at the feet, without any initial tensing of muscles element. At the end of the progressive relaxation, I ask for feedback with an implication that she will probably have noticed spontaneous alteration in sensory awareness of body size, shape, weight, and temperature, e.g., "What do you notice now about the apparent weight of the body?" (Note the use of the words "what"–nonspecific, "now"–implying there has already been a change, "apparent"–acknowledging that it is not factual, and the use of "the" body, promoting dissociation, as opposed to using "your" body.) This feedback is useful for providing trance ratification. A posthypnotic truism suggestion is then given that if she can dramatically change her perceptions of such unalterable physical characteristics, then she will also have the ability to change her thoughts, feelings, emotions, and responses. Then perhaps add "these are far easier to change than the physical characteristics that you have already changed."

The first session finishes with clear instruction in a virtually foolproof and often very impressive simple self–hypnosis technique using clasped hands index finger attraction (see page 174). This allows the woman to place herself in self-hypnosis in less than sixty seconds. A direct suggestion can be given that when she is recognizably in trance, she will have the ability to simply imagine herself in some future setting, being well and leading the sort of life she would like to live. I ask that she imagines this future scenario in the present tense and that when the session finishes, the memory of this image will be a past event. I frequently say that this mixture of past, present, and future images confuses the brain and, within reason, can allow the image to become a self-fulfilling prophecy as the subconscious seeks ways to achieve the image. This approach is commonly used in sports hypnosis. The woman is instructed to practice this technique daily and return in one week. I tell her that I will expect her to be able to put herself in and out of a trance at will when she returns for her next lesson the following week. More than 98 percent of women return for the next session.

During the next week, the woman is bound to think positively about her first experience of hypnosis. She learns, with each practice session, that she can put herself into a relaxed frame of mind that is called "trance." In trance, she may experience her body very differently. This feeling of unreality, or altered feeling of reality, makes it easier to accept that she can imagine other future scenarios such as wellness or fertility that might have seemed unreasonable to the conscious mind of the present.

The Second Session

The second most useful generic hypnotic technique after relaxation is to teach a version of creating a unique special place of bliss. The concept of creating a personal "Special Place" that can be utilized in therapeutic hypnosis or self-hypnosis is relatively common practice in modern hypnosis. Some therapists prefer to describe the contents of such a special place in detail while others prefer that the client chooses his/her own imagery for their special place. The version that I frequently use, I call the "Special Place of Bliss" imagery (SPBI). It goes far beyond the basic hypnotic theme of having a "Special Place" as simply a place of psychological safety. The SPBI is a generic technique that can be employed by a wide range of people presenting with an even larger variety of problems. It allows people to be able to symbolically put all of their worries and problems, at least temporarily, off to one side. The SPBI allows the client absolute privacy and autonomy of choice at several points. The role of the therapist in the SPBI is to facilitate the client to cooperate in the therapy process and in fact to largely become his or her own therapist. This is accomplished by supplying very minimal structure that only has meaning when the client personalizes the imagery and gives it specific meaning. I have used the SPBI with over a thousand individual hypnosis clients in recent years. Feedback from clients suggests that the impact of the SPBI imagery experience is often extremely powerful and therapeutic. Using the SPBI in self-hypnosis regularly, or even at times on a single occasion, can often resolve the presenting problem of a large number of clients. This is particularly the case if one of the presenting complaints is that of initiatory insomnia. The SPBI can also permit resolution of other issues that have not even been discussed or presented and of which the therapist has no knowledge. I have even used the SPBI to good effected in a case where the client asked if I could help her deal with a problem without her having to disclose any details to me about what her problem was. The SPBI empowers the client to have and take considerable control over the impact of his or her problems. While I disagree with using set scripts as a magical incantation, you may find this particular script useful if you are faced with a woman presenting for hypnosis with a gynecological problem and you are unsure of what to say that may be therapeutic. This would apply especially if you have limited medical knowledge of the pathophysiology of her condition. . . .

Some key points of the SPBI are noted in the following transcript:

"I'd like you to imagine walking along a corridor. As you walk along the corridor there are doors that lead off to the left and to the right. Doors to the left and doors to the right. *(This repetition of the words left and to the right facilitates some horizontal to-and-fro eye movements.) (This corridor with the doors can be used in later sessions if you wish for a variety of other therapeutic purposes.)*

"At the end of the corridor you'll find a door. *(nonspecific direct suggestion)*

"A very inviting sort of door. *(still nonspecific but friendly—some doors may have had a bad connotation for the client)*

"You can decide for yourself the size and shape of the door..... *(first direct offer of choice)*

"And tell me, what color is the door that you see?................ *(wait for verbalized answer)*

"Is the *(insert color)* door plain or is it paneled? *(more choices)*

"Does the door have a handle?

(If yes) "Is the handle on the left or on the right?

"Now look very closely, does the door seem to open inwards or outwards?

(The specific answers to the above questions do not usually matter but sometimes the chosen color, shape, or other characteristic of the door are of great significance to the person. Answering these simple questions establish-

es that the subject is actively visualizing a particular door. Inviting someone to see a door of their choosing is a fairly easy visualization request. Inability to see a door suggests there is a problem of some sort, usually inadequate preparation.) (Do NOT proceed further with this imagery until the subject can confidently see a specific door.)

"You may be wondering about this door. About what lies behind the door. In a few minutes you will discover that behind the door is a special place. Your very own special place. A special place that your imagination is already creating for you. It is a special place. A special place of bliss. Absolute bliss! Now bliss is an old fashioned word. It's not used much nowadays. Let me be quite clear about what I mean by bliss. Bliss, as you know, is a state of mind. Bliss is the absence of negativities. The absence of worries, the absence of problems, concerns, difficulties, traumas, upsets, and anxieties. *(This should cover far more than just the presenting complaint)*

"But bliss is far more than that. As well as the absence of negativities, bliss is also the positive presence of such concepts as freedom, peace, comfort, joy, happiness, relaxation, and rest. Absolute pleasure . . . sheer . . . bliss. So, in order to experience a sense of bliss, then we have to be able, at least on a temporary basis, to put all of our problems and worries off to one side. So, on your back you will find a backpack. Take the backpack off and place it in front of you. As you open the backpack, you will find inside it a collection of stones. Notice how the stones are somewhat flat, but rounded and smooth, rather like the sort of stones you might find on the bed of a river or a rocky beach. . . .

"Do you see the stones? *(Wait for confirmation.)*

"Since this is hypnosis, then these stones are symbolic stones. The stones symbolically represent all of your problems. Each stone represents a problem. The stones represent all of the problems that you have in your mind. Some of the stones represent the problems of now, the present. The issues and concerns that are on your mind now, today, this very day.

"But almost certainly there are stones about the past. And the past includes yesterday, last week, last month, last year, ten years ago, many years ago. All the way back to your earliest memories of childhood.

"And some stones represent the future. How can this be since the future hasn't happened yet. Well, these are what I call the "What if?" stones. Anticipation stones. Some people carry around stones that represent their worries about what might happen in the future. What could go wrong. What might not change. These stones represent possibilities. Sometimes quite remote possibilities that ought to be pebbles. But some people carry them around like rocks of probabilities. Or even as huge boulders of near certainties. *(Every possibility, past, present, and future is covered.)*

(Privacy guarantee)

"And because these stones represent every problem, not just the ones that you have told me about. I want to make one thing very clear. Some of these issues may be very personal. Therefore, for this reason, I want to assure you that this next part of the exercise will be carried out in total and absolute privacy. Now by total and absolute privacy I don't simply mean the usual confidentiality that you can expect and will, of course, receive from a doctor. No, I actually mean far more than that. By total and absolute privacy, I mean that I want you to do the next part of the exercise entirely inside your own head, in silence. What this means is that only you will ever know what particular issues these stones mean to you. Let me be absolutely clear. I will never, ever, ask you to talk about the meaning of any of your stones.

"Only you will ever know how many stones are in the backpack. Again I will never, ever ask you to talk about the number of stones. And perhaps most importantly of all, only you will ever know the weight of each particular stone. Obviously, the weight of each stone relates to the weight of the problem. Again I will never, ever ask you to talk about the weight of any of the stones. Now, is that guarantee of privacy completely understood? *(Wait for confirmation of understanding.)*

"Now look at the stones in the backpack. In a few moments, I will give you the signal to start unloading the backpack. Remember that it's quite safe to do so. These are flat stones. They can't roll away.

"When it's time, I want you to look at the top stone. It will probably have a label on it. To let you know what problem it represents. I want you to read the label and identify the problem. Then, briefly, to feel the weight of the stone and then simply place it down on the floor beside the (insert chosen color) door. Then turn to the back pack and identify the next stone, feel the weight of that stone and then put it down beside the door. Then when you have taken the time you need to completely empty your backpack you can let me know that it is empty by raising your right thumb in the air. Are those instructions clear? *(Wait for confirmation)*

"Then turn to the backpack and now start unloading all your problems . . . stone by stone . . . issue by issue . . . problem by problem . . . till the bag is completely empty. Take all the time you need.

(Give the person time to empty their stones. A few useful interjections every so often can be helpful, e.g.)

"Some of the stones are the ones you expected to find there. Others might be a bit of a surprise.

"Some of the stones may be heavier than you had expected. Some may be surprisingly light.

"Some of the stones may have been there for a long time.

"Some problems can have three stones. One for the past, how you used to feel about the problem. One for how it affects you now. And one for the future about anxieties you might have about what it may be like in the future.

"Take your time. Take all the time you need.

"Stone by stone.

"Some stones may have lost their labels. Hard to remember what those stones represent. If they are from the past, then they represent something that happened, but you've forgotten the details. But they still have weight so take them out and put them down by the door. If it's a shiny new stone of the future without a label then that is just generalized worry . . . about nothing specifically.

"Some people have lots of stones. Others only a few.

"Some people collect pebbles. Each pebble is small. Not very heavy. But a lot of pebbles together can add up to a lot of weight. Each pebble is too small for a label. Too time consuming to unload individually . . . so you can just tip any pebbles out at the end. You can just raise your thumb when the backpack is emptied. *(Wait till the thumb eventually rises then proceed to the next phase.)*

"Now turn to the door. Put your hand on the handle and go through the doorway into your special place. The door closes behind you. Feel the sense of bliss in this special place. Feel the sense of freedom. Look around at the place you find yourself. It may well surprise you. It may be quite different from what you were expecting. Can you describe what this place is like to me? *(Utilize whatever imagery is reported and interpret it in the most blissful way. Let the person spend a few minutes experiencing a sense of blissfulness.)*

"Now go back to the door and leave the special place of bliss. You can always go back there. Perhaps go there to experience bliss every day. I like to start my day with experiencing a few moments of bliss.

"Now look at the stones lying beside the door. These stones represent all your problems. Past, present, and even future. Only you know what these stones represent. Only you know how many stones there are. At this point, you might like me to wave a magic wand and make all the problems disappear. But that's not possible. That would be fantasy. This is reality. And you know in reality there are some things that cannot change. You cannot change the past. You cannot change one minute of the past. Not even one second of the past. In the same way, you cannot change the stones. You cannot change the size, the shape, the color, the texture or the number of stones. These cannot be changed. But there is one really important change that you can make. You can change the location of the stones.

"If you want, for some or even perhaps for all of the stones, you could choose to leave the stones lying there. What difference would that make? They would still have the same size, shape, color, and texture as before. But if you left the problems lying there, on the floor, you would not be able to feel the weight of the stones anymore. This would turn each problem into a technicality. Just a mere technicality. On the floor you wouldn't be able to experience the feeling of weight any more. . . . Does that make sense*? (Wait for confirmation and give clarification if needed.)*

"On the other hand, if for whatever reason, for your journey through life, you feel a need to carry some or even all of the stones as a sense of burden, then feel free to pick up some or even all of the stones and put them in the backpack. The essential ingredient of a burden is the weight, the load. To experience the problems as a burden you need to be able to feel the weight of the problem. . . . Does that make sense? . . . Can you appreciate the difference between a burden and a technicality? . . . Then carefully make your choice for each stone. You don't have to decide for the rest of your life. Just for today. Are there any stones that you don't need to carry as a burden for the rest of today. If so you can leave them there. It's quite safe. Remember that these are flat stones. They won't roll away. They will still be the same problems. They will still have the same size, the same shape, the same texture, the same color. But you can now choose whether to carry the weight. You cannot change your problems. But you can choose whether you regard them as burdens or as technicalities. . . . Take your time and choose. It's awesome. . . . When you have made your choice for the location of each stone, again in absolute privacy, then you can let me know by raising your thumb once more. *(Wait till thumb rises)*

"Now put the backpack on your back and start walking along the corridor. See the doors to the right and the left. As you walk back along the corridor you may see some stones on the floor. Some people are what I call "habitual stone picker-uppers." No one is born a stone picker-upper. You have to learn it. Usually you learn it from a parent. Often a mother stone picker-upper. 'Oh, there's a stone. Be a good girl and pick it up.' Lots of messages from childhood about 'ought to' and 'should.' I'm sure you know what I mean by that.

"But some people with a lot of stones in their backpack are not habitual stone picker-uppers. They are usually very generous people. Often they are warm hearted and giving. But it's as if they go through life with their backpacks wide open and this allows other people, or events, but usually other people to dump some of their stones into our backpack. And I'm sure you know what I mean by that.

"There was a song in the 1960s sung by The Seekers and by The Byrds called 'Turn, Turn, Turn.' You might remember the song. 'There is a season, turn, turn, turn. . . .' There is a line in the song that says 'A time for laying down of stones, a time for gathering stones together.' The words of the song were not written in the sixties but in fact come from the Bible. I don't know what the original writer meant by those words, but I suspect that the original writer would be happy with this modern day use of these words. You can choose when it is your time to lay down your stones. Each day you can lay down your stones and experience your special place of bliss. Each day you can choose the location of your stones. Even if you feel obliged to pick them all up again, you can still be refreshed by spending time in the place of bliss. Some days you may be able to leave all the stones lying on the floor as mere technicalities. On those days, you can then start your day with a clear mind. You can repeat this exercise in your own time as often as you wish. I like to do it each morning. Each time will be different. You will learn something new each time you do. You can start each day with a sense of bliss. You can lay down your stones. In so doing you can convert your burdens into technicalities.

"But for now just gradually reorient yourself to this room and to this time. Hear the noises around you more clearly and when you are ready just gradually open your eyes and come out of trance. How was that?"

(Do NOT ask about the stones—Respect their total and absolute privacy. Keep your word!)

.... I am sometimes asked to treat people who either cannot afford the cost of personal therapy or are unable to travel to Wellington or New Zealand. To help these people, I have recorded a generic version of the first two sessions described above that is available on audiotape (McCarthy, 1998). Subsequently, in letters from far-flung areas and countries, people whom I have never met in person have reported deriving considerable benefit from listening to the instructions on the tape.

The Third Session and Beyond

The third and subsequent sessions are when the hypnotic individualization that is appropriate to each woman and her presenting problem takes place. By now the woman has become accustomed to using self-hypnosis and many women report that they have developed a new and hopefully better perspective on their problem by "unloading their stones." Even at this stage, where the session content varies considerably from woman to woman, I still like to opt to use a fairly generic and still nonspecific technique that can be used across a variety of clinical situations to teach a specific hypnotic skill or exercise. Opting to go for a very specific therapeutic message early on in the therapeutic relationship is risky. There is an all-or-nothing aspect to symptom specific suggestions that is best avoided by keeping the intended result of the session still artfully vague and using a technique that the woman will be able to use successfully to some extent. Success is important. Success breeds success!

I tend to see most women for only about six therapeutic sessions. I would expect some useful change within the first two to three sessions.

One session often includes the Erickson quote given earlier. If the woman has a symptom of pelvic pain associated with her particular problem, then I will usually use one session to teach the glove anesthesia technique and dissociation and hyperassociation exercise as described in the obstetric section of this chapter. Another useful session for many women (the 4-finger technique) is particularly helpful for women who claim to have very little time to devote to practicing self-hypnosis. This consists of teaching her a useful anchoring technique to associate touching her right thumb against the tip of her right index finger with a memory of loving or being loved. The thumb then touches the tip of the middle finger and is associated with a memory of listening to the sound of being paid a compliment. The right thumb then touches the tip of the ring finger and this is associated with the memory of "honest tiredness" from some physical exertion such as a long walk. The right thumb then touches the little finger and this retrieves a vision of something that was aesthetically beautiful to behold. I then simply state that the index finger memory of the loving experience is stored in the left frontal lobe. The memory of the sound of the compliment is stored in the left temporal lobe. The kinesthetic memory is stored in the base of the brain and the visual memory is stored in the occipital lobe at the rear of the brain. (This is analogous to the limbic-hypothalamic explanation given earlier.) In theory, with each finger having a top, middle, and bottom as well as a back and a front, then the right hand can store up to 24 memories, 6 loving memories, 6 compliments, 6 times of healthy tiredness, and 6 wonderful sights. The left hand can store "memories of the future" that have a similar theme as the right hand, but obviously these are made up and imagined. I state that accessing all parts of the brain, front, side, base, and rear can swamp any unwanted thoughts of today. The unwanted thoughts of today can be matched and overloaded with good thoughts of the past and the future. This technique uses both hands and both hemispheres and thus gives less space for unwanted thoughts. The exercise can be carried out in a mere 60 seconds: 10 seconds to enter trance, 5 seconds for each of the eight fingers, and then 10 seconds to exit from trance. The excuse of never having time does not apply to such brief self-therapy that takes one minute and can be repeated several times a day with or even without eye closure.

There are a huge variety of other generic metaphors that can be utilized in the other sessions depending on what skills the woman is deficient in to assist her in reaching her goals. It is important to have a whole host of other techniques and metaphors at your disposal. Michael Yapko's book *Trancework* (1990) explains how to design a therapeutic metaphor.

For a woman who often puts herself down and has a low self-esteem due to the impact of her "inner critic," I could opt to use what I call the "silly voices" routine. This consists of asking her to think a common negative thought that she often has about herself. She is then instructed to listen carefully not to the "verbals" of the negative thought but to the "vocals." She is then instructed to project the voice to her shoulder and imagine the exact same words but now delivered in a silly voice. If the believability of the thought is reduced, then she knows that the validity of the comment is enhanced or diminished by the tone of the voice. She can choose to change the voice of her inner critic. If this is useful, I then ask her to imagine the voice coming from her armpit. This often causes her to smile and to say that the negative thought seems ridiculous and lacking in believability now.

The basic principle of hypnosis therapy in gynecology, however, is simply to teach more and more skills until the woman realizes that she is not helpless and that she can use her mind to modify her awareness so that she is able to cope with her presenting symptoms more easily. This might mean that her problem goes away or that she can cope with her problem better. As stated earlier, on average, I see women with gynecological problems for perhaps only six or seven 30-minute sessions in total and then see them for follow up at perhaps one month and three months later. A word of caution, however, from personal experience: the more rapidly that a woman responds to therapy, the more hypnotizable she tends to be and the more carefully you have to follow her up, as her chances of relapse are higher given the risk of reexposure to negative surroundings.

Given the rich psyche-soma link of gynecology, there is surprisingly comparatively little research and literature written about the use of hypnosis in gynecology when contrasted with its use in general medicine or other surgery. There is even less material that I can confidently recommend being worth reading. The approach that I use with hypnosis for gynecology is based on recent concepts of psychoneuroimmunology (PNI) and the role of the subconscious that were not readily available to earlier writers. David Cheek's ideas, based on considerable experience, about the use of hypnosis in gynecology (Rossi &

Cheek, 1994) certainly make interesting and challenging reading. You will have to decide for yourself, however, how applicable such ideas are to your own practice and beliefs.

The classical American hypnosis textbook *Handbook of Hypnotic Suggestions and Metaphors (Ed. Hammond)* (1990), for instance, has only a few specific mentions of gynecology, and the most common presenting gynecological problem that I see, endometriosis, is not even mentioned at all. This book does, however, have some extremely useful insights into a range of hypnosis techniques in the treatment of female sexual dysfunction that have been contributed chiefly by the editor himself who has extensive experience in both hypnosis and sex therapy. Please note that Hammond (1990) strongly emphasizes that sex therapy is no place for the hypnotic tyro, however.

Let me finish with a plea for more research and clinical use of hypnosis in gynecology. Even if you are a hypnotic tyro, you are unlikely to do much harm by teaching a women how to be more in control of her thoughts, feelings, emotions, and responses and how to be able to choose to alter her interpretation of reality in a positive way. If her problematic gynecological symptom or condition is due to a powerful signal from her subconscious, then a useful final comment to make in trance to end the first phase of therapy is the following. "Your symptom(s) may well *have been* a warning signal. If, however, everything that can be done, and should be done, has been done, then you may well find that there is no longer a need for the same signal." In many cases the preinduction session and all the sessions thereafter are all aimed ultimately at delivering this crucial empowering message with it's inferred posthypnotic suggestion. It's not a command, it's only a suggestion after all–and suggestion is what hypnosis is all about.

REFERENCES

Beck, A., Rush, J., Shaw, B., & Emery, G. (1979). *Cognitive therapy of depression.* New York: Guilford Press.

Beck, N.C., & Hall, D. (1978). Natural childbirth–A review and analysis. *Obstetrics and Gynecology, 52:* 371–379.

Blackburn, I. M., & Davidson, K.M. (1995). *Cognitive therapy for depression and anxiety: A practitioners guide.* Oxford: Blackwell Scientific Publications.

Brann, L.R., & Guzvica, S.A. (1987). Comparison of hypnosis with conventional relaxation for antenatal and intrapartum use: A feasibility study in general practice. *Journal of the Royal College of General Practitioners, 37*: 437–440.

Burrows, G.D. (1978). *Obstetrics, gynaecology and psychiatry.* Melbourne: Hi Impact Press.

Charles, A.G., Norr, K.L., Block, C.R., Meyering, S., & Meyers, P. (1978). Obstetric and psychological effects of psycho-prophylactic preparation for childbirth. *American Journal of Obstetrics and Gynecology, 131*: 44–52.

Coble, P.A., Reynolds, C.F., & Kupfer, et al. (1994). Childbearing in women with and without a history of affective disorder: Psychiatric symptomatology. *Comprehensive Psychiatry, 35*(3): 205–214.

Collins English Dictionary, Third Edition. (1991). Glasgow: Harper Collins, 1991.

Cox, J.L., Murray, D., & Chapman, G. (1993). A controlled study of the onset, duration and prevalence of postnatal major depressive disorder. *British Journal of Psychiatry, 163*: 27–31.

Davenport-Slack, B. (1975). A comparative evaluation of obstetrical hypnosis and antenatal childbirth education. *International Journal of Clinical and Experimental Hypnosis, 12*: 266.

Erickson, M.H., Hershman, S., & Secter, I. (1961). *The practical application of medical and dental hypnosis.* New York: Brunner/Mazel.

Fee, A.F., & Reilly, R.R. (1982). Hypnosis in obstetrics: A review of techniques. *Journal of the American Society of Psychosomatic Dentistry and Medicine, 29*:17–29.

Grant, V.J. (1998). *Maternal personality, evolution and the sex ratio: Do mothers control the sex of the infant?* London and New York: Routledge.

Haley, J. (1973). *Uncommon therapy, the psychiatric techniques of Milton H. Erickson M.D.* New York: W.W.Norton.

Hammond, D.C. (Ed.)(1990). *Handbook of hypnotic suggestions and metaphors.* New York: W.W. Norton.

Harmon, T.M., Hynan, M.T., & Tyre, T.E. (1990). Improved obstetric outcomes using hypnotic analgesia and skill mastery combined with childbirth education. *Journal of Consulting and Clinical Psychology, 58*, 5: 525–530.

Hilgard, E. R. (1979). Hypnosis in the treatment of pain. In G. D. Burrows et al. (Eds.), *Handbook of hypnosis and psychosomatic medicine.* New York: Elsevier.

Hilgard, E. R., & Hilgard, J. R. (1994). *Hypnosis in the relief of pain.* Los Altos, CA: W. Kauffman, Inc.

Jenkins, M.W., & Pritchard, M.H. (1993). Hypnosis: practical applications and theoretical considerations in normal labor. *British Journal of Obstetrics and Gynaecology, 100*: 221-22.

McCarthy, P. (1998). Hypnosis in obstetrics. *Australian Journal of Clinical and Experimental Hypnosis,* Vol.26 No.1: 35–42.

McCarthy, P. (1998). *Mind and body relaxation. Relaxation hypnosis, self-hypnosis and how to create your own special place of bliss.* (audio-tape). Dr. P. McCarthy, Wellington.

Oster, M. I. (1994). Psychological preparation for labor and delivery using hypnosis. *American Journal of Clinical Hypnosis, 37*:12–21.

Reynolds, J.L. (1997). Post-traumatic stress disorder after childbirth: The phenomenon of traumatic birth. *Canadian Medical Association Journal, 156*: 831–5.

Rossi, E.L., & Cheek, D.B. (1994). *Mind-body therapy–methods of ideodynamic healing in hypnosis.* New York: W.W. Norton.

Saner, G., & Oster, M. I. (1997). Obstetric hypnosis: Two case studies. *Australian Journal of Clinical Hypnosis, 37*:74–79.

Schaper, A.M., Rooney, B.L., Kay, N.R. & Silva, P.D. (1994). Use of the Edinburgh Postnatal Major Depressive Disorder Scale to identify postpartum Major Depressive Disorder in a clinical setting. *Journal of Reproductive Medicine, 39*(8), 620–624.

Seligman, M. (1990). *Learned Optimism.* New York, Knopf.

Stone, P., & Burrows, G.D. (1980). Hypnosis and obstetrics. In G.D. Burrows & L. Dennerstein (Eds.), *Handbook of hypnosis and psychosomatic medicine.* New York: Elsevier Press.

Waxman, D. (1989). *Hartland's medical and dental hypnosis* (3rd ed., pp. 384–411). London: Bailliere Tindall.

Werner, W.E.F., Schauble, P.G., & Knudson, M.S. (1982). An argument for the revival of hypnosis in obstetrics. *American Journal of Clinical Hypnosis, 24*, 149–171.

Yapko, M.D. (1990). *Trancework: An introduction to the practice of clinical hypnosis* (2nd ed.). New York: Brunner/Mazel.

Yapko, M.D. (1994). *Suggestions of abuse: True and false memories of childhood sexual trauma.* New York: Simon & Shuster.

Yapko, M.D. (1992). *Hypnosis and the treatment of depressions: Strategies for change.* New York: Brunner/Mazel.

Yapko, M.D. (1997). *Breaking the patterns of depression.* New York: Doubleday.

Zeig, J. (1990). *Seeding in brief therapy.* J. Zeig & S. Gilligan (Eds.) New York: Brunner/Mazel, 1990.

Chapter 10

PERSPECTIVES FROM PHYSICIAN/PATIENTS

KAREN OLNESS

INTRODUCTION

Hypnosis has been reported as sole anesthesia for surgery since 1843 when Elliotson and Braid wrote papers about its use. Shortly thereafter, chemical anesthesia came into general use and hypnosis was used infrequently. During this century, there have been reports from time to time about the use of hypnosis as sole anesthesia (Victor, August, Levitan); a number of videotapes demonstrating this are in the archives of the American Society of Clinical Hypnosis and the Minnesota Society of Clinical Hypnosis. They demonstrate hypnosis as sole anesthesia for cesarean section, nasal surgery, thyroidectomy, hip surgery, and abdominal surgery. In general, hypnosis has been used when patients are intolerant of specific anesthetics or prefer not to have chemical anesthesia. The latter was true with respect to the three case histories described in this paper. Two of them involve myself, and one involves a physician who was one of my trainees. The procedures took place in 1987, 1988, and in 1997. One was videotaped and has been used in hypnosis teaching for the past decade. The purpose of publishing these case histories is to document that hypnosis does provide an option for persons scheduled to have surgery, and also to emphasize that research in this area is needed.

First Surgery–Repair of "Gamekeeper's Thumb" (KO)

In 1968, I first learned cyberphysiologic strategies for relaxation and pain control. I realized that I had, in fact, used something similar for control of discomfort in the dental chair for many years. As a child, I learned that by focusing intensely on the image and feeling of participating in a tennis game, I felt comfortable and required no local anesthesia. Later, as I began to teach children skills in self-hypnosis, I was amazed to learn how quickly they could acquire pain management skills, and I resolved to develop these myself. During the early 1970s, I practiced regularly (once daily) for two months to learn to control incoming uncomfortable sensations such as needle sticks.

As the years went by, I had no particular occasion, to use my control except in the dental chair. On one occasion, when I had an inlay done with no anesthesia, except my own, I felt very comfortable in the dental office. The procedure was completed. I paid my bill and stepped out on the sidewalk. Immediately, I was overwhelmed with a dreadful pain in my right jaw. I realized that I had given myself a suggestion to be comfortable in the dentist's office; therefore, I had to return to the waiting room, sit down for a few minutes, and change the suggestion for comfort to last as long as necessary until the discomfort from the procedure had faded away. I imagined myself in a favorite, safe, comfortable place, found my mental control switch for the nerves to the affected tooth, turned it off, and then told myself that the switch would remain off until all discomfort from the tooth had faded away.

I had long stated that if I should need general anesthesia, I would make an effort to use my own pain control. The opportunity came when I sustained a Gamekeeper's thumb injury while skiing. It was necessary to reattach ligaments supporting my left thumb. The orthopedist was inexperienced in having a patient who refused chemical anesthesia. He was somewhat anxious about this, and I did my best to be reassuring to him.

My preparation consisted of listening to a relaxing meditation tape for 30 minutes prior to the procedure and placing myself mentally in a very comfortable favorite place, i.e., the farm on which I grew up. The entire procedure was videotaped and my EEG was also monitored. I received psychological support from two colleagues who were in the operating room during the procedure. One was running the camera and EEG, and the other gave me hypnotic suggestions. The suggestions were general, relating to feeling safe, comfortable, and in control. I also focused on remaining in my favorite place. At times my colleague would ask, "Where are you now?" I would respond with a description of what I was seeing or doing, and I felt that it was difficult for me to talk. Once I said, "I am playing with my cat." He asked, "Is this a male or female cat?" I replied, "No one knows." He said, "The cat knows." I had a strong feeling of support from friends, which was very important, and I felt comfortable.

One of my colleagues played music that I did not particularly like–synthesizer music–but I was not much aware of the music until I later heard it while watching the videotape. During the surgery, I had a brief period of cognitive dissonance when the surgeon said, "now we will be drilling." As I relaxed "on the farm," I anticipated the sound of the drill, but none came. After a few minutes, I thought that the drilling must have occurred and somehow I had missed it. Shortly thereafter, I imagined myself in a sports car about to drive down the highway near the farm. There was a sudden whine from the drill. Immediately I incorporated into my mental processing and imagined that I was stepping forcefully on the accelerator. Later, when viewing the videotape, I noted that my right foot moved down when the drilling began.

I also had some cognitive dissonance when I felt something wet on my left hand near the end of the procedure. I wondered if it was blood, and I wondered if I should turn off the bleeding. I thought that extra blood flow might not be necessary to bring healing substances to my left hand and thumb. I later learned that the wetness came from the saline flushes. In retrospect, I wish I had been told what was happening. When the surgeon said he was through, I just gradually opened my eyes, enjoying the feeling of pleasant relaxation. I sat up and the surgeon said, "Well, I must say, I'm impressed."

I was very happy as I left the operating room. I had lunch with a friend and spent the afternoon working. During the evening, I was aware of some aching in my left thumb area. I controlled this with self-hypnosis. I took no medication before, during, or after the procedure.

Case History 2–Removal of Breast Lump (KO)

In January, 1997, I had a normal mammogram. In March, 1997, during a routine exam, a right breast lump was detected. Following an ultrasound, a surgeon did a needle biopsy, interpreted as epithelial hyperplasia. Following this, the surgeon recommended excision of the lump. A second ultrasound was done and second opinion obtained which confirmed the recommendation. The lumpectomy was scheduled for early May. The surgeon was open to doing the procedure without sedation or general anesthesia.

I prepared an audiotape for myself with suggestions for comfort, turning off pain signals to the right breast area, the right amount of bleeding, and healing. This included suggestions such as "Enjoy being comfortable and peaceful, knowing you can allow the right amount of bleeding for healing and cleansing, bringing immune substances to the area in just the right amount." "Turn down the dimmer switch controlling the nerve signals from the right breast to nearly off. You may feel the surgery as a gentle, healing touch." I taped the verbal suggestions over piano music played by my husband. I listened to the tape three times before the day of surgery.

After the preoperative examination by a resident anesthesiologist, however, I became concerned that my intention to use self-hypnosis might be sabotaged. While the resident expressed interest in self-hypnosis, it was clear that he knew nothing about it and I recognized that inadvertent negative or skeptical statements in the operating room might be detrimental to the hypnotic process, even in an experienced subject. So I called an anesthesiologist who was positive about the use of hypnosis to ask if he might speak to the OR staff on the day of my surgery. Fortunately, he was in charge of the OR on that day and he stopped by in the pre-op suite where I waited. He himself placed the intracath, a "security" measure. Although I had not allowed placement of intravenous access for my first surgery, I did not object this time. I trusted my colleague and knew that he wanted to place the intracath in case general anesthesia or other medication was needed during the procedure. Two nurses inquired if I would like to have a pre-op sedative. I quietly refused and listened to my tape.

I was relaxed and comfortable when I was wheeled into the operating room. My pulse was 62 and my blood pressure 100/60. I listened to the tape and the timing seemed almost perfect with respect to the time of the procedure. Only one aspect bothered me. I was tipped to the right on the operating table. Although there were straps to hold me, I had the constant feeling that I was sliding toward the right and off the table. So I braced myself with my left leg which felt very fatigued at the conclusion of the procedure. By the time of the excision, the lump had become much smaller. The pathologist read it as negative. The procedure took 20 minutes. I was amazed how well timed my tape was in terms of suggestions regarding pain, bleeding, and healing. I felt that was about 20 minutes.

When the surgery ended, I was wheeled into the post-op area, taken immediately to get dressed, and then walked home to eat breakfast. By noon, I was working in my office. Once again, I felt enormously pleased to have used my self-hypnosis successfully and to be spared the post-op problems associated with anesthesia.

Case History 3–Inguinal Herniorrhaphy (RK)*

In December, 1987, while doing squats, weight lifting 315 lbs., I felt a shift in my lower abdomen while at the bottom of a squat and on the way up. It wasn't painful; it didn't hurt. It was just a peculiar kind of shift. I wasn't even sure if my weight belt had slid or exactly what had taken place. In subsequent days, while Christmas shopping and walking around malls, my left hip would hurt. It was really peculiar–the interior thigh and left hip. I found that if I sat down for awhile it would go away. I kept thinking, "well gee, I deal with all these patients with osteoarthritis; this must be what hip pain feels like," and so on. I decided that I would do more squats just to make sure that my legs were nice and strong so that when I developed my arthritic conditions, whatever they might be, I would be fit and able to take it all in stride. The discomfort got more and more annoying. It was peculiar, however, that after prolonged walking it hurt sometimes and sometimes didn't.

In January, I developed a cough. With this cough I saw bulging in my lower abdomen, in the inguinal area. "Ah-ha, I have got an inguinal hernia which is giving me a nerve entrapment sort of syndrome in referring the pain out to the hip and anterior thigh. I saw a colleague of mine who was a surgeon. He was also a fellow college graduate and graduated from the same medical school as I. I can't particularly say that we knew each other. I just respected him and felt that he would be a good surgical person to examine me and confirm my diagnosis, and I would trust his opinion regarding treatment. He examined me one day at work and said, "Yes, you've got an inguinal hernia, there's no doubt." He examined the other side; that was solid, firm and fine. He then asked, "When do you want to have surgery?" Well, I figured I would give myself a month to prepare, so I told him

---

*This is a summary from a dictation done in September, 1988.

that February 11, 1988 would work out fine. I then contacted an anesthesiologist who I heard had used hypnosis in the past, but had moved away from it because it took too much time. However, at least he was an anesthesiologist who understood hypnosis.

I told the anesthesiologist what I wanted to do. He understood completely and was excited and interested in helping me. The anesthesiologist said that we had to practice hypnosis, induction of anesthesia at least once, and then he wanted me practicing on a regular basis. He came to my office one day. He had me draw two circles, in pen, on my left forearm, and when I was relaxed, he told me to point to the circle that I wanted anesthetized. I selected and pointed to my circle. He proceeded to lift up that area and stuck a hypodermic needle through it; something we have all seen done before. It's no big deal. I wasn't quite sure if I was "gutting" it out or was it actually painless. I felt him do it. I can't say that it hurt. It was endurable. It really didn't seem to have any effect on me. What did have an effect on me was when he told me to open my eyes and look at it, which I proceeded to do and then proceeded to faint. He then knew exactly what type of subject he was dealing with; somebody who was squeamish as hell! My entire staff was wondering what was going on. He asked my staff for smelling salts. I came out looking white as a sheet. He had also given me a hypnotic suggestion. I practiced this on a regular basis, once or twice daily, anesthetizing some part of my body that touched the inguinal area or just thinking of anesthetizing the inguinal area directly, using whatever modality I wanted to use that we both knew were available. I would spend 30 to 45 minutes laying on my bed, relaxing myself and developing various images for anesthetizing the area.

Now the day of surgery approached. I had asked the Department of Education if it would be videotaped. The surgeon said he would take care of it, which he did not. There was a tiny bit of aversion that I had about having this on videotape. I felt it would perhaps jeopardize my performance, rather than enhance it. So, I asked for a video once and then let the fates fall as they may.

It was the day surgery was set for. We checked in smoothly. We went up to the day surgery rooms where I undressed. They told me that I would be going in at about 7:00 AM. I had arranged beforehand that the physical therapist would come to me in the recovery room and tens (transcutaneous nerve stimulation) would be put across the incision, and the OR sterilized pads would be there. The physical therapist would hook up the tens units in the recovery room for me to use for incisional discomfort if needed. There was also the definite understanding among myself, the anesthesiologist, and the surgeon that if the repair was at all jeopardized by my inability to relax, the surgeon was to inform the anesthesiologist, and he would give me chemical anesthesia. And, if the anesthesiologist, at any point, was uncertain whether or not I was having any discomfort or pain, he had the right to go ahead. I had given myself the instructions to need the least amount of anesthesia and that recovery from anesthesia would be fine if needed. And so a nice safety net was established before the surgery.

Thirty minutes before surgery, they pulled me from the room, which was great! Now I could concentrate on relaxing and not on my wife. I figured I needed to know and do nothing, that the medical system was set up enough that they would tell me what to do and I would respond. That was it. I didn't need to look at the people around me or at anything, so I closed my eyes. I had no pre-op medication. I went down to the elevator; waited in a room outside the OR. They took me down to the OR, I put myself on the table. The whole time my eyes were closed; I was quiet. Nobody greeted me or spoke to me.

Once on the operating table, my arms were strapped down, the blood pressure cuff put on, an IV started. The first IV attempt was in my left arm and was unsuccessful. I figured if anything was going to happen to me, it was going to happen now. He chose another spot, and got a good stick. Therefore, I had the opportunity to practice pain control right there. He did not anesthetize the area, and put a huge IV in. He strapped my arms down. I liked the feel of the blood pressure cuff inflating and I decided that I was going to use that as a distraction technique as well. I used the washing of the inguinal area as a signal to deepen my trance. At home, I had practiced that I would feel the cold washing and shaving of the inguinal area and use this as a deepening technique. I had also given myself instructions to use the feeling of pressing down the adhesive material (which is used to pick up the loose hair after shaving) for deepening. Obviously, you can feel the pressure, but you can't feel the sensation, so that was an adjunct deepening technique for anesthetizing the area. When they put the drapes over me, I used that as a deepening technique. The anesthesiologist was talking to me the whole time. The surgeon came into the room. I felt his presence. I did not listen to his words. I only listened to the anesthesiologist. I could hear my heart rate on the monitor. I felt the beginning of the incision. I forgot all of my planned techniques and said, "You've got to do something now," in my head, and I projected my consciousness out to the three story parking ramp and watched the people come to work. I visualized the snow. I have very fond memories about the snowfall, the coziness of people in their coats, people coming into work, and me this silent observer watching all of this, warm and cozy. That's simply what I did – a technique I hadn't practiced at all. I just displaced myself out of the top of my head, sitting on the edge of the parking ramp. But there's no seat there and there's this little disembodied individual watching the people come to work and smiling and happy about watching that. Surgery was proceeding. I wasn't feeling anything. I was feeling things, but there was no pain. Upon hearing my heart rate increasing on the monitor, I became aware that my leg was jumping. I could hear the bovie and knew they were stopping bleeders. I could feel the ground pad and my whole left leg jumping each time the surgeon bovied the bleeder. I knew that I had to get this under control now or they were going to give me general anesthesia. At that time my eyes were open. I could see the anesthesiologist learning forward, and he actually did talk to me. It was like I was the outside observer, and yet I knew I was in my body. I was in a dissociated state. I could see him lean forward to my left ear and he said, "I'll give you a few moments to deepen your trance." And then, the next thing I heard was the bovie, and my leg was still, which was amazing. Surgery proceeded and I heard my heart rate going up again, and I'm saying, "They're not going to allow that. They're going to think you are in pain. You're going to have to slow your heart rate. You've got to bring things under control." And sure enough, on the basis of that, the blood pressure was stable. The anesthesiologist again leaned forward and said, "He's manipulating your intestines. There may be come discomfort. I'm going to give you some oxygen." I thought, "Great! He's probably going to mix it with something." I could see the black mask going over and the oxygen felt cool. It was very interesting and I didn't feel anything other than that. I felt the oxygen and breathed it. No big deal. Surgery continued and at this point the surgeon said he was tempted to give me a local, but he gave me no local. He had 7 cc. of lidocaine that he had drawn up that he was going to infiltrate around the cord if my heart rate did not go down. He wasn't going to have the anesthesiologist give me general anesthesia because the surgery was nearly completed. He didn't use the lidocaine and he started to complete the repair. I felt him suture the individual layers, almost with glee. With each little prick, silence. I had a great sense of comfort with the perception of stitching. I knew he was suturing me and had closed the incision. He then cleaned off the area with gauze. I felt his warm hand over the area and he said, "Well, we did it." I started to get off the table and he said, "Wait a minute! I've got to pull these drapes off and dress the wound. Did you forget that this needs to be done?" They then dressed the wound. At this point, I still hadn't opened my eyes. They dressed the wound, brought in the gurney. I transferred myself to the gurney and didn't feel a thing. I didn't hurt at all when moving. The anesthesiologist told me that just before dressing he gave me a regional block and put the tens pads on. I went to the recovery room and couldn't feel anything. I was wide awake in the recovery room and drove the nurses crazy because I scoured my chart for any evidence that he gave me anesthesia with the oxygen. I was talking to my friends, who were surgeons coming into the OR and wondering what I was doing there and why I was awake, why I wasn't vomiting my guts out, rolling and turning and shivering like the other patients around me. By protocol, they had to keep me an hour in the recovery room. I read the chart. The anesthesiologist came out of surgery saying I did a great job and I should be proud of myself. I practically jumped off the cot and put him up against the wall and said, "Did you give me anything?" and he said, "No, no, no. The surgery was done and we gave you a regional block after the surgery because we all know you fully intend to go to work tomorrow, although we would advise you to stay at home. We want you to be comfortable. The block will last maybe 24 hours at best." He said, "Just use your relaxation techniques to heighten the ability of the block to work." I then left recovery and returned to the day surgery rooms. I've eaten without vomiting. I drank something without vomiting, but I hadn't urinated. They weren't going to discharge me until I had voided. I had a couple liters of fluid. I drank four diet Cokes. I can't even feel my bladder. So I shut off the tens unit, and I could feel the fullness of my bladder. I got out of bed, went into the bathroom, and voided. I decided the tens unit was not helpful because it was anesthetizing my bladder. I decided I would not go home with it. I returned to the bed and was waiting for the nurse to come and say I could get dressed and leave. My wife said, "Tell me what went on." She had no idea that I was planning to have surgery without anesthesia. I didn't want to tell her in advance. I didn't want any performance anxiety and I didn't want anyone else wondering how I was going to do or worrying about my choice or anything like that. I started to describe to her the surgery just as I have done on this tape. When I got to the incision part and the feeling of the incision and what I did, I felt myself growing queasy. I punched the light and said, "Oh, oh." Nurses came rushing in, flipped me over, opened my IV site and ask my wife what was happening. I had done everything right and they were about to release me. I explained to them I just felt squeamish when I described my surgery. So it was an amazing event even in recovery. The ride home was comfortable. I walked up the stairs to my bed. I had a little problem getting into a comfortable position in bed. I took aspirin, which they had advised against because of bleeding, but I told myself that I wasn't going to bleed, I wasn't going to swell and aspirin helped with the discomfort at this point. I slept reasonably well. I was stiff and awkward when I got out of bed the next morning, but I did get dressed and went to work. I put in a six hour day and it was a Friday. I came home about 2:00 in the afternoon and rested until 5:00. I got dressed in my tuxedo and went to a benefit dinner. I had someone else drive me, both to work and to downtown. My surgeon was at the same event. He proceeded to praise me for what I had done and chastised me for being at the dinner. My only very painful event at the benefit dinner was that I had a sip of a Manhattan. I can't handle liquor very well, and this was very strong. I coughed, and that did hurt.

About four days after the surgery, the repair was tight and I could feel tension from the inguinal to the ilioinguinal ligament. I could feel the tension of the fascia between those two areas, as if cellophane tightened over the bony prominences and ligaments. I started using visualization to thank it for being tight, to communicate to the other side that it remain tight, that my abdominal musculature would be tight and strong, that I would shortly return to lifting again, that I would never develop a hernia on the other side, and that it would be firm and solid.

I resumed my workouts in a week and generally increased their length and intensity. At eight weeks, I had resumed all my triathlon training activities, swimming, biking, and running. In August, I did the Chicago Triathlon with 3,000 others and finished it in two hours and 50 minutes. My previous best time was two hours and 45 minutes. I had a very good run compared to the previous year and a reasonable bike, and my weakest was my swim.

That's the story of my inguinal hernia repair. If I can do it, anybody can do it. What happened amazes me, but it's not my skill. I focused my interest and took that focused intention, practiced it, and then I let go of it and let God help. I don't care how corny it sounds; it's what happened to me.

Comments

It is clear that the hypnotic strategy used for these procedures was a combination of dissociation and direct suggestions for eliminating pain signals. Both of us were comfortable during the surgical procedures and had a positive sense of accomplishment at their conclusions.

Review of the experiences emphasizes how important it is for the surgeon or anesthesiologist to prepare the patient and to tell the patient, who may have eyes closed and not seem to be paying attention, if there are changes in plans or procedures. Paradoxically, although the patient dissociates, he or she also wants to know exactly what is going on.

The experiences described document the two levels of functioning in a hypnotic state. We were dissociated and yet able to think about what was happening with respect to the surgery. The failure of the surgeons to explain that there was a problem attaching a drill bit, and to note that they were flushing the wound with saline might contribute to a "lightening" of the trance and to a less effective experience. There are few surgeons in the United States who are knowledgeable about hypnosis and use it in their practices. This is a disadvantage for the patient who would like to use hypnosis. The patient must provide education and persuasion about his or her ability to be comfortable without local or general anesthesia. We were both physicians who were able to do this. It is less likely that a nonphysician would be successful in persuading the surgeon.

In summary, this chapter describes use of hypnosis as sole anesthesia by two physicians. They avoided side effects of chemical anesthesia and enjoyed the adjunct benefit of a wonderful sense of control.

EPILOGUE

Considering the vast amount of research which has been done during the past 30 years, only part of which has been cited in the preceding chapters, one wonders what will become known in the field of hypnosis and its application during the next 30 years. The technology, the availability of the computer and the increased speed of communication should contribute to an even greater knowledge and appreciation of hypnosis. More will be known about the intricate relationships of body and mind, and their interdependence. It will be up to the healthcare profession to get involved, and become familiar with the value and the advantages which this medical modality brings. Then it will be possible, among other things, to help every human being to prevent the ill effects upon their psychological as well as physiological parameters, which are created by the tremendous apprehension, stress, and anxiety which they experience prior to surgery and other painful procedures. It is my hope that the circulation of this and other books, which will follow, will speed the acceptance of hypnosis, and its use by all who are privileged to take care of surgical patients.

AUTHOR INDEX

A

Abraham, H. A., xii
Abramson, M., 85
Adams, P. G., 104
Adcock, R. J., 44, 131
Aitken, H., 60, 71
Aitkenhead, A. R., 71, 85
Albert, L. H., 38
Anderson, J. A. D., 40
Andolsek, K., 158
Atkinson, G., 16
Auerbach, S. M., 65
August, 212

B

Bagby, E., 17
Bakan, P., 68
Baker, J. M., xii
Baker, K. H., xvi, 60
Banyai, E., 13
Barabasz, A., xiii, 75
Barabasz, M., 75
Barber, J., xiii, 4, 8, 19, 38, 66, 81, 109, 133
Bartlett, E. E., xiv, 64, 67, 102
Bartlett, M., 4, 7
Basker, M. A., 40
Bates, B. L., 106
Battit, G. E., 64
Beale, I. L., 39
Beck, A., 163, 179, 181, 182
Beck, N. C., 163
Beecher, H. K., 33, 38, 83
Behrendt, D. M., 64, 85
Bennett, H. L., xvi, 3, 60, 64, 72, 79, 85, 102, 121
Bensen, V. B., 68, 82, 102
Benson, D. R., xvi, 3, 60, 64, 72, 79
Benson, H., 13

Bernheim, H., 7
Berstein, M. R., 100
Bienias, J. L., 105
Bierman, S. F., 158
Bishay, E. G., 72
Bjerring, P., 108
Black, P. H., 60
Blackburn, I. M., 181
Blankfield, R. P., xiii, 85
Blass, M. H., 100
Blass, N., 107
Bleeker, E. R., xvi
Block, C. R., 163
Bloom, L. R., 85
Boltwood, M. D., 132
Bombardier, G. H., 44, 131
Bonke, B., 60
Borrows, A., 121
Botta, S. A., 101
Bowen, D. E., 100
Bowers, K. S., xi–xiii, 5, 16, 17, 37, 38
Braid, J., xi, 212
Brann, L. R., 164
Breckenridge, J. L., 71
Breuer, J., 7
Bridger, A. A., 19.
Brooke, R. I., 40
Brown, D. E., 4
Brown, J. M., 4
Brunn, J. T., 59
Brunnquell, D., 139, 160
Burnam, M. A., 83
Burns, G. L., 131
Burrows, G. D., 39, G. D., 163
Bystedt, H., 3, 72

C

Callen, K. E., 39

Campanella, G., 108
Casiglia, E., 64
Cedercreutz, 40
Chapman, C. R., 3, 38, 43, 83
Chapman, L. G., 131
Charcot, J. M., 7
Charles, A. G., 163
Chaves, J. F., 4, 72
Cheek, D. B., xii, 4, 58, 59, 61, 63, 67, 68, 70–72, 74–75, 79, 106–8, 120, 121, 126, 127, 130, 135, 148, 188, 208
Ciottone, R. A., 57
Clarke, J. C., 12, 20
Clawson, T. A., Jr., 79, 101
Cloquet, J., 99
Coble, P. A., 179
Cocke, J. R., 86, 100
Coe, W. C., xiii, 4, 67
Cohen, F., 85
Colgan, S. M., 39
Council, J. R., xiii
Covino, N. A., xvi
Cox, J. L., 179
Crasilneck, H. B., xii, 12, 20, 39, 51, 100, 121
Crawford, H. J., 13, 24
Culbert, T., 60
Cummings, C., 40

D

d'Hnin de Cuvillers, Baron, xi
Dalton, J., 40
Dane, J. R., xiii, 86
Darwin, C., 190
Davenport-Slack, B., 163
Davidson, K. M., 181
Davis, H. S., 60
de Puysegur, Marquis, xi
Diamond, M. J., 4
Dillon, M., xvi, 60
Disbrow, E. A., 85
Doberneck, R. C., 102
Domangue, B. B., 3, 38, 41
Donaldson, G. W., 40
Dot, S. G., xii
Doubt, T. J., 64
Downie, C. F. A., 60, 71
Dubin, L. L., 3, 73

DuHamel, K., 66
Duke, J., 68
Dumas, R. G., 64
DuMaurier, G., 7

E

Edmonston, W. E., 12
Egbert, L. D., 64, 102
Eich, E., 121
Eimer, B. E., 41, 49
Eli, I., 100
Elkins, G. R., xiv
Ellenberger, H. F., 7
Elliotson, J., 99, 212
Elton, D., 39
Enqvist, B., 3, 59, 64, 72, 102
Eremin, O., 75
Erickson, M. H., 4, 13, 20, 58, 65, 75, 132, 157, 163, 186, 187
Esdaile, J., xii, xiv, 3, 94, 99, 100, 114
Evans, B. J., xiii, 37–41, 43, 48, 64
Evans, C., 71, 81, 85
Evans, F. G., 59
Evans, F. J., 4–7, 9, 10, 13, 15, 16, 17, 24, 34, 35
Everett, J. J., 131
Ewin, D. M., xii, 38, 62, 63, 68, 102, 131

F

Faragher, E. B., 39
Farvolden, P., xiii
Faymonville, M. E., 84
Fee, A. F., 163
Fellows, B. J., 86
Fernandez, A., 100
Ficher, 64
Finer, 39
Fisher, R., 84
Fisher, S., 66
Fissette, J., 84
Fitsh, W., 60
Fordyce, W. E., 33, 41, 44
Fortin, F., 64
Frank, J. D., 9
Frank, K. A., 85
Frank, R. G., 39
Frankel, F. H., xii, 19

Frederick, C., 130
Fredericks, L. E., xv, xvi, 64, 66, 68, 73, 100
Freeman, A., 41, 49
Freud, S., 7
Fromm, E., xiii, 4

G

Gainer, M. J., 39
Gauld, A., xiii, 94
Gekoski, W. L., 37, 38
Genest, M., 33, 41
Gerton, M. I., xi
Giannini, J. A., 60
Goebel, R. A., 100, 107
Gold, P. E., 57
Goldman, L., 64
Goldstein, E., 38
Goodell, H., 131
Gottheil, E., 85
Grabowska, M. J., 72
Grant, V. J., 190
Gravitz, M. A., xi, 64
Greenberg, L. M., 71
Greenfield, L., 85
Greenleaf, M., 66
Grevert, 38
Gruen, W., 104
Guerra, F., 120
Guzvica, S. A., 164
Gwynn, M., 67

H

Haanen, H. C. M., 39
Hacket, T. P., 64, 85
Hagens, J. H., 64
Haley, J., 157, 186, 187
Halfen, D., 107
Hall, D., 163
Hall, H. H., xvi, 122
Hall, J. A., 12, 20, 51
Hammer, A. G., 4 , 7
Hammond, D. C., 12, 20, 50, 51, 108, 209
Harbaugh, T. E., 104
Harmon, T. M., 165, 166
Harper, D. C., 83
Hart, R. R., 85
Hekster, G. B., 39

Heller, S. S., 85
Heron, W. T., 85
Hershman, S., 163
Heyman, D. J., 64
Heys, S. D., 75
Hilgard, E. R., xi–xiii, 3–5, 7, 13, 15, 16, 19, 24, 34, 35, 38, 75, 83, 100, 104, 105, 163, 166
Hilgard, J. R., 3, 35, 38, 75, 100, 104, 163
Hind, M., 84
Hoenderdos, H. T. W., 39
Holroyd, J., 39
Hop, W. C., J., 39
Horne, R. L., 17
Hoskovee, J., 121
Houge, D. R., 66
Houghton, L. A., 64
Howard, J. F., 71
Hull, C. L., 4, 10, 19
Hunter Farr, J., 101
Hunter, M. E., 12, 20, 51
Hutchings, D., 102, 103
Hynan, M. T., 165, 166

I

Iwamoto, K., 104

J

Jackson, J. A., 12, 20
Jacobson, E., 13
James, F. R., 39
Jenkins, M. T., 100
Jenkins, M. W., 164
Johnson, G. M., 121
Johnson, L. S., 104
Johnson, V. C., 75
Johnston, M., 58
Jones, J., 71
Jones, J. G., 60
Joris, J., 84
Joyce, J. S., 84

K

Kenny, G. N. C., 60, 71
Kessler, R., xiii, 65, 86
Kihlstrom, J. F., xiii, 59, 120, 121

King, B. J., xiii
Kirouac, S., 64
Kirsch, I., xi, 105
Klein, K. B., 64, 75
Kleinhauz, M., 81, 100, 128
Kline, M., xii
Knox, V. J., 37, 38
Knudson, M. S., 163
Kohen, D. P., 139, 138, 141, 142, 151, 156–58, 160
Kolouch, F. T., 57, 103
Konieczko, K., 71
Konow, 3
Konow, L., 72
Kornfield, D. S., 85
Kostka, M., 101
Kraemer, H. C., 85
Kroger, W. S., 100
Kuiken, D. A., xvi, 3, 60, 64, 72, 79
Kurtz, R., 105
Kuttner, L., 139, 141, 151, 160
Kvaal, S., 104

L

LaBaw, W. L., 73
Lafontaine, C., xii
Lambert, S. A., 142, 143
Lamy, M., 84
Lang, E. V., 84, 97, 135
Large, R. G., 34, 39
Lazarus, H. R., 64
Lazarus, R. S., 85
LeCron, L., 108
Lee, 72
Leonard, R. C., 64
Letendre, A. J., 57
Levey, A. B., 64
Levinson, B. W., 59, 79, 120
Levitan, A. A., xii, 100, 104, 212
Linden, J. H., xi
Lingley, J. F., 57
Linssen, A. C., 40
Liu, W. H., 85
Livnay, S., 108
Lowenstein, L. N., 104
Lucas, O. N., 72
Lynn, S. J., xiii, 4, 81, 104, 130

M

Macdonald, H., 104
MacDonald, J. T., 40
Magaw, A., 68
Mallee, C., 39
Mambourg, P. H., 84
Mann, T., 7
Mare, C., 104
Margolis, C. J., 3, 38, 39, 41, 73
Mark, J. B., 71
Markowsky, P. A., 16
Marvin, J. A., 131
Mason, A. A., 100
Mathews, A., 58
McCarthy, P., 166, 175, 206
McCauley, J. D., 39
McCranie, E. J., 100
McDonald, H., 83
McGlashan, T. H., 34, 35
McGrath, P. A., 40
McLaughlin, D. M., 37, 38
McLintock, T. T. C., 60, 71
Meichenbaum, D., 33, 37, 41
Melmand, G., 140
Melzack, R. V., 38, 39, 49
Mesmer, F. A., xi, xiv, 3, 6, 99
Meyering, S., 163
Meyers, P., 163
Mialle, xi
Miaskowski, C., 66
Millar, K., 60, 121
Miller, N. E., 24, 37, 38, 64
Millet, J., 60, 79, 103
Minchoff, B., xvi, 60
Mishkin, M., 75
Mitchell, W. A., 6
Mittleman, K. D., 64
Moore, L. E., 72
Morgan, A. H., 19, 83, 104
Morris, D. M., 100, 107
Moskowitz, R., 85
Munglani, R., 60

N

Nathan, M. G., 100
Nathan, R., 107
Norr, K. L., 163

Novik, B., 158

O

O'Connell, D. N., 19
Ogg, T. W., 64
Olness, K., 40, 41, 60, 76, 128, 138, 139, 141, 142, 157
Orne, E. C., 7, 24, 59, 105
Orne, M. T., xiii, 7–9, 12, 14, 15, 17, 19, 24, 34, 35, 59
Ornstein, R., xiii
Osler, Sir W., 128
Oster, M. I., 163
Owings, J. T., 85

P

Patterson, D. R., 44, 131
Pearson, R. E., 59, 64, 67, 71, 79, 102, 106
Peebles, M. J., 121
Pennebaker, J. W., 83
Perry, C., 38, 39
Pert, C., 58, 68, 76
Peter, B., 70
Peterson, L., 140
Peterson, P., 67
Petri, H., 75
Phillips, M., 130
Price, D. D., xv, 132
Prior, A., 39
Pritchard, M. H., 164
Pulos, L., 99

Q

Questad, K. A., 132
Quirk, M. E., 57

R

Rasmussen, 141
Rasputin, 72
Rausch, V., 101
Reich, P., 64, 79
Reilly, R. R., 163
Reynolds, J. L., 169
Rhue, J. W., xiii, 4
Richardson, P., 71, 81, 85
Ridgeway, V., 58

Rodger, B. P., xiv, 64
Roediger, L., 84
Rogers, M., 64, 79
Rossi, E. L., 4, 13, 58, 67, 68, 70–72, 74, 75, 107, 108, 121, 127, 130, 135, 148, 188
Rudy, T. E., 49
Ruiz, O. R., 100

S

Sacerdote, P., 3, 38
Salmon, P., 57
Sampiman, R., 100
Sarbin, T. R., 4
Sauer, C., 163
Scaba, S., 135
Scagnelli, J., 110
Schachter, D. L., 59
Schaper, A. M., 179
Scharffer, M. A., 83
Schauble, P. G., 163
Schneck, J., xii
Schoenberger, 66
Schultz, J., 112
Schultz-Stubner, S., 95
Schwarcz, B. E., 100
Schwartz, H., 104
Scott, D. L., 104, 120
Secter, I., 163
Segal, D., 104
Seibel, L. J., 140
Seligman, M., 179–82
Shapiro, S., 3, 73
Shigitomi, C., 140
Shor, R. E., xiii, 7, 16, 19, 34, 105
Shum, K., 37, 38
Silverberg, E. L., 85
Sime, A. M., 58
Sivec, H., xiii, 104
Smith, P., 75, 128
Smitz, P., 60
Sobel, D. S., xiii
Solomon, Z., 81, 128
Spanos, N. P., xiii, 4, 19
Spiegel, D., xii, 19, 20, 24, 38, 40, 64, 75, 84, 85, 96, 105, 107
Spiegel, H., 8, 19, 20, 23, 24, 96, 105, 107, 133
Spielerger, C. D., 57
Spinhoven, P., 40

Stam, H. J., 39
Standen, P. J., 85
Stanley, G. V., 39
Stanley, R. O., xiii, 64
Stern, D. B., 24
Sternbach, R. A., 31, 33, 41, 44, 46
Sternberg, D. B., 57
Stevens, 72
Stone, P., 163
Strobel, 39
Surman, O. S., 64, 85
Swade, R. H., 79, 101
Sweeney, B. P., 84
Swersky-Saechetti, T., 73
Syrjala, K. L., 40

T

Tan, L. T., 33
Tan, M. Y.-C., 33
Teitelbaum, M., 100
Tellegen, A., 16
Tennenbaum, S. J., 105
Terwiel, J. P., 39
Thelen, M. H., 39
Thompson, K. F., 101, 159, 160
Tinterow, M. M., 95
Tobias, J. D., 141
Torem, M. S., 74, 107, 135
Trustman, R., 121
Tucker, K. R., 104
Turk, D. C., 33, 41, 49
Turndorf, H., 64
Turner, J. A., 3, 38, 43, 83
Tyre, T. E., 165, 166

U

Uden, D. L., 40, 60
Unesthal, L. E., 25, 50

V

vanDyck, R., 40
VanDyke, P. B., 102, 104
vanRomunde, L. K. J., 39
Verhage, F., 60
Victor, 212
Vingoe, F. J., 13

Virnelli, 104
Visintainer, M. A., 140

W

Wagstaff, G. F., 4, 35
Wain, H. J., 79
Walker, L. G., 75
Wall, V. J., xiv
Walling, D. P., xii
Walsh, S. L., 108
Warner, D., 75
Watkins, J. G., xii, 104
Waxman, D., 163
Weekes, J. R., xiii
Weinberger, N. M., 57
Weitzenhoffer, A. M., 4, 7, 10, 12, 19, 20, 105, 120
Welsh, 64
Werner, W. E. F., 163
Whiting, P. H., 75
Whorwell, P. J., 39, 64
Wickramasekera, I., 83
Wiesner, S. L., 72
Willard, R. R., 39
Williams, A. R., 84
Wolfe, L., 60, 79, 102, 103
Wolfer, J. A., 140
Wolff, H. G., 131
Wollman, L., 104
Woodruff, M., 100
Woody, E., xiii

Y

Yapko, M. D., 58, 63, 169, 179, 181, 182, 208

Z

Zachariae, R., 108
Zeig, J., 196
Zimmerman, J., 65
Zitman, F. G., 40
Zwaveling, A., 60

SUBJECT INDEX

A

Absorptive experiences, xi (*see also* Relaxation)
Acupuncture vs. hypnosis, 37
Acute pain, 31–38, 43–45 (*see also* Chronic pain; Pain management)
   acute vs. chronic pain differences, 31–38
   anxiety management, 43–44
Adler School of Professional Psychology, xiii
Age progression, 176
Age regression, 12, 198
Altered state of awareness, xi, 58–59, 65, 67, 70, 95
Altered state of consciousness, xiii, 4, 6, 65 (*see also* Special process theories)
American Society of Clinical and Experimental Hypnosis, xii, 20
Amnesia, posthypnotic, 15, 61–68, 79, 101–3, 175
Analgesia, 12, 49, 52, 66, 97, 108–10, 134, 177–78
   glove analgesia, 12, 49, 52, 66, 97, 108–10, 177–78, 207
Anesthesia, general and hypnosis, 57–87, 176–78
   altered state of awareness, xi, 58–59, 65, 67, 70, 95
   anxiety, stress' impact on postoperative recovery, 57–58, 66–84
   autonomic nervous system responses, 64, 58
   critically ill and altered state of consciousness, xi, 58, 120
   epinephrine: memory fixation and anxiety triggers, 57
   fear and postoperative recovery, 58
   information processing while under anesthesia, 59, 107
   interoperative suggestion, 59–63
   loss of control perception, 57, 65
   major surgery and altered state, xi, 58–59, 65, 67, 70, 95
   medical procedures and anxiety, 57
   postoperative suggestion and recovery, 64–68, 149
   preoperative psychological state and recovery, 57, 100
   surgery, anxiety, and stress, 57–58, 66–84
   surgical anesthesia and information processing, 59–63, 107
   therapeutic suggestions, 59
Anesthesia, hypnotic, 99–114 (*see also* Hypnoanesthesia)
   absence of medical side effects, 95, 100
   application, 104
   benefits to physiology 100–3
   general anesthesia reversion, 111
   historic overview of sole use, 99–101
   implementation, 104–7
      glove analgesia, 12, 49, 52, 66, 97, 108–10, 207
      ideomotor signaling, 63, 108
      susceptibility assessment, 104–5
   physiological benefits, 100–3
   prerequisites for practitioner, 106–7, 114
      electroencephalogram, 104
      neurosurgery, 104
   procedure, 107–14
      glove analgesia, 12, 49, 52, 66, 97, 108–10, 207
      patient preparation and training, 109–11
      self-hypnosis, 110
Anesthesia, regional and hypnosis, 94–98
   altered state of awareness, 95
   deepening techniques, 97, 178, 219 (*see also* Rapid indirect induction techniques)

glove analgesia, 12, 49, 52, 66, 97, 108, 109, 207
hypnosis and absence of side effects, 95, 97
inadequate spinal or epidural, 95
    anxiety level and suggestibility, 95
    induction by eye fixation on ceiling, 96
        procedure, 96
    induction by eye roll relaxation, 96, 105, 107, 133
        procedure, 96
intravenous anesthesia, side effects, 95, 97
managed care time constraints in patient/physician relationship, 96
Monitored Anesthesia Care, 94
Anesthesiologist's role in allaying fear, 63–64
    patient evaluation re anxiety, 68
        gaze direction, 68
        informed consent and preop suggestions, 70
        physiological responses, 68, 76–78
        presurgery sedation, 74
        relaxation, dissociation suggestions, 69
        role of praise for patient suggestion, 71
        transference and countertransference, 71
    preparation of patient: pre-surgery, 68–78
    ——suggestions, 70–76
    ——induction of anesthesia, 78
    ——during surgery, 79
    ——emergence from anesthesia, 80–81
    ——recovery room, 81–84
    ——pain sensations, 82–84
Anorexia, brain tissue loss and hypnotizability, 191
Anger and chronic pain, 43–45
    key questions to evaluating pain patients, 47
Animal magnetism, xi, xiv
Anxiety
    anticipatory fear, 44, 102
    depression and pain behavior, 44
    helplessness and pain behavior, 44
    key questions to evaluating pain patients, 47
    pain stimulation, 43–45, 83
    psychological meaning, 83, 100
    reduction, 82–84
    surgery anticipation, 65–84, 102
Applications of hypnosis, xii
    unusual medical situations, xii
Arthritic pain, 24–26
Autonomic functions, xv
Awareness, altered states of, xi, 5, 58–59, 65, 67, 70, 95, 126

B

Biofeedback vs. hypnosis, 38, 39
Bleeding
    hemophiliacs, xvi, 3, 72–73
    influence of hypnotic suggestion, xvi, 43, 64, 72, 78–80, 101
    surgery, xvi, 3, 64, 72, 78–80, 101
Bone marrow transplants, 40, 41
Bowel functioning, 73, 82, 84, 102, 113
Braid, James and hypnosis terminology, xi
Bulimia nervosa, brain tissue loss and hypnotizability, 191
Burns, xii, 38, 44, 102, 130–33, 13
    interruption of burn progression, 130–31
    role of hypnosis in intervention, 130–32

C

Cancer, xii, xvi, 3, 38, 39, 41–43
    hypnosis and pain management, 41–43
        chemotherapy side effects, 41
        imagery techniques, 43
        medication reduction, 41–43
        nausea, 41, 102
        self-hypnotic procedures, 43
            cancer remission caution, 43
            long-term effectiveness, 43
Case studies and physician perspectives
    medical modalities and hypnosis, 38–41
    physician surgery
        breast lumpectomy,
        gatekeeper's thumb, 212–14
        inguinal herniorrhaphy, 216–22
    Vietnam land mine injury, 32–33
Catalepsy, 176
Children and surgery, 138–61
    belief in child's ability to communicate, 139
    case examples, 142, 143–46, 147–48, 151–54, 155
    child needs, 139–61
        anesthesia induction, 146

details of procedure and purpose explanation, 139–40
during surgery, 148–51
ego strengthening, 149–50, 156
emergency room, 156–60
preoperative tours, 140
psychological preparation, 140–41
rapport with practitioner, 141, 156, 158
regional anesthesia, 154–56
role playing, 140
hypnotic approach determined by
connecting communicatively with child, 138–39
developmental level, 138, 139
individual needs, 138
learning style, 138
personal interests 138
pain management, 151
pediatric anesthesiology, 138
pediatric intensive care unit, 151–54
postoperative suggestion, 149–51
switches, framing and using, 150–51, 155
terminology of pain, reframing, 141, 157–58
Chronic pain, xvi, 3, 13–15, 31–53 (*see also* Acute pain; Pain management)
acute vs. chronic pain differences, 31–38, 43–45
clinical assessment, 45–49
confrontational assessment style, 46
four direct pain summary questions, 46–48
faulty communication loop, 18
hypnotic techniques, 49–51
imagery techniques, 13–14, 49
key questions to evaluating pain patients, 47
pain management and hypnosis, 31–53 (*see also* Pain management)
positive, negative hallucinations, 15
Co-consciousness and multiple cognitive pathways, 5
Cognitive dimension, 12–15
imagery, 13–14, 49
positive, negative hallucinations, 15
relaxation, 12–13, 49
trance logic, 14–15
Conception aid, xii, 186
Consciousness (*see also* Unconscious)
comatose and information encoding, 60, 107, 120–21
critically ill and information encoding, 60, 107, 120–21
hearing and imprinting information, 60, 107, 120–21
ideomotor movement response procedure, 24–26, 52, 60, 63, 121
levels of, 5
surgical anesthesia and information processing, 59–60, 107, 120–21
Contagion compliance in hypnotic performance, 6–7
Critically ill and altered state of consciousness, xi, 58, 120

D

Death, fears of, 74
Deepening techniques, 97, 178, 219 (*see also* Rapid indirect induction techniques)
Defense mechanisms
altered state of awareness, xi, 5, 59, 65, 67, 70, 95, 126
Definitions
Altered state theorists, xiii
APA, xi
Barabasz, xiii
Kihlstrom, xiii
overview, 4–18
social-psychological theorists, xiii
Dental patients, 5, 38–39, 138
Depression and pain stimulation, 43–45
anticipatory fear, 44
depression and pain behavior, 44
helplessness and pain behavior, 44
key questions to evaluating pain patients, 47
Depression, postpartum, 178–82 (*see also* Obstetrics and gynecology)
attributional style analysis, 180–82
permanency, 180
impermanent for bad, 180
personal, 180
impersonal bad, 180
personal good, 180
pervasive, 180
nonpervasive bad, 181
pervasive good, 181
cognitive thinking, reframing, 179
incidence, 178

overview of symptoms, 179
Post Natal Major Depressive Disorder Scale, 179
psychosocial factors, 179
skill-based approach, 181
    characteristics of training program (list), 181
Differential arm levitation hypnotic technique procedure, 21–23
Dissociation
    age regression, 15, 198
    analgesia, 12, 15, 49, 52, 66, 97, 108, 109, 135
    and hypnosis, 15–18, 49, 52, 66, 97, 108, 109, 135
        deep hypnosis, 15
    and obstetrics, 178
    and pain relief, 15
    anesthesia, 15
    multiple personality, 17
    negative hallucinations, 15
    posthypnotic amnesia, 15, 61–68, 79, 101–3, 176–78
    posthypnotic suggestion, 15, 58, 65, 73, 82, 84, 102, 113, 119, 176–82
    posttraumatic stress syndrome, 17, 169
        from obstetric labor process 169–71
    triggers, 18, 52
        dissociation, 176–77
Dissociative experiences, xi, xiii, 5

E

EEG patterns, 13
    hypnosis, 13
    sleep, 13
Emergency room, 126–36
    altered state of awareness, xi, 58–59, 65, 67, 70, 95, 103, 113, 126, 127
    burn patients, 130–31, 138 (see also Burns)
    communications styles
        fully informed, confident, 127–29
        negative suggestions, 127
        nonverbal, 127, 128
    fight or flight and rapid induction, 133
    heightened state of suggestibility, 103, 113, 126, 128
    negative belief system into positive one, 130
    pain management, 129
    pediatric patients, 156–60
    permissive hypnotic approach, 130
Emesis, 40, 82, 102, 113, 119
Esdaile, James and surgical hypnosis, xiv, 3
    pain, control of, 3
    surgical application and patient survival, 3
Eye gaze direction and hypnotic capacity, 68
Eye roll relaxation hypnotic procedure, 23–24, 43, 96, 105, 107, 133
Expectation, 5–10, 97, 105, 106
    hypnotist behavior, 9, 106–7
    placebo response, 9–10

F

Fibromyalgia, 39, 44
Fictional literature's depiction of hypnosis, 7
Four-finger technique, 207

G

Gastric secretions, 64
Glove analgesia, 12, 49, 52, 66, 97, 108–10, 207
Goal-directed strivings, xiii
Gynecology (see Obstetrics and gynecology)

H

Hallucinations, 176
Handbook of Hypnotic Suggestions and Metaphors, 209
Happens to, rather than result of doing, xiii, 6
Harvard Group Scale of Hypnotic Susceptibility, 19, 105
Headaches, 12, 39, 40, 44, 76
    migraine, 39, 40, 76
    tension, 40
Healer-to-healee relationship, xi, 4
Heart rate and rhythm, xvi (see also Deepening techniques; Self-hypnosis)
Hemophilia, xvi, 3, 72–72 (see also Bleeding)
Hidden observers, 104
Hint and Run technique, 65
Historic hypnotic experiences
    Aesculapian rituals, xi
    animal magnetism, xi, xiv
    artificial somnambulism, xi

Delphic Oracle consultation, xi
hypnoanesthesia, xii
sleep temples, xi
Historic introduction, 3–4
Hospital residency programs and hypnosis training, xi, 86–87, 222–23
Hypnoanesthesia, 100–114
    application, 104
        electroencephalogram, 104
        neurosurgery, 104
    general anesthesia reversion, 111
    implementation, 104–7
        glove analgesia, 12, 49, 52, 66, 97, 108–10
        ideomotor signaling, 63, 108, 121
        susceptibility assessment, 104–5
    physiological benefits, 100–3
    prerequisites for practitioner, 106–7, 114
    procedure, 107–14
        glove analgesia, 12, 49, 52, 66, 97, 108–10
        patient preparation and training, 109–11
        self-hypnosis, 110
Hypnosis
    absence of medical side effects, 95, 100
    benefits, 100–3
    APA definition, xi
    historic introduction, 3–4
    induction, 20–26 (see also Hypnotic induction)
    measurement, 18–20 (see also Hypnotic measurement)
    overview, 4–18
    placebo response, 9–10
    special process vs. socio-psychological theories, xiii, 4, 6
    trance markers, 9
Hypnosis and
    anxiety/stress, 57–87
    clinical applications, surgical, 57–87, 100–14
    cognitive-behavioral approaches, xiii, 4, 6, 12–15
    direct v. indirect, 52
    ego strengthening, 52, 104, 133, 149, 150, 178
    memory, 57–87
    pain control, 4, 49–51, 102 (see also Glove analgesia; Self-hypnosis)
    rehabilitation, 52, 102
    relaxation inductions, xi, 8, 20–26, 52, 97, 104–14
    screening tests, 7, 14, 18–20, 49
    surgery, 57–87, 99–114
        recovery outcomes 84–86, 100
    surgical recovery, 57–87, 100–3
    tailoring to patient, 49–50, 100
    time distortion, 63, 102–3
Hypnotic ability and dissociation, 15–18
Hypnotic behavior dimensions, 5–18
    cognition, 12–15, 26 (see also Cognitive dimension)
        imagery, 13–14
        positive, negative hallucinations, 15
        relaxation, xi, 8, 12–13, 20–26, 49, 52, 69, 97, 104–41, 133
        trance logic, 14–15
    dissociation, 15–18, 26, 104 (see also Dissociation)
    expectation, faith, belief, 5–10, 26, 97, 105, 106 (see also Expectation)
    suggestion, 10–12, 26, 105–6 (see also Suggestion)
Hypnotic induction, xi, 8, 20–26, 97, 104–14
    differential arm levitation procedure, 21–23
    eye roll relaxation procedure, 23–24, 105, 107, 133
    ideomotor movement response procedure, 24–26, 52, 60, 63, 121
    imagery and metaphors, 13–14, 66, 97
    prerequisites for practitioner, 106–7
Hypnotic Induction Profile, 19, 105
Hypnotic measurement, 18–20
    screening, 18–20
    series of graded suggestions, 18–19
Hypnotic susceptibility, 13, 16, 66–68
    and postoperative recovery, 66
Hypnotic trance, 174–75
    hypnotist's behavior, 9
    prerequisites for practitioner, 106–7
    superstitious behavior, 9
Hysterectomy word derivation, 182–83
Hysteria, 7

I

Ideomotor movement response procedure, 24–26, 52, 60, 63, 108, 121, 175

IgA levels and hypnotic induction, 60, 76
Imagery, 13–14, 66, 97, 107–8, 175–76
    deepening techniques, 66, 97, 108
    guided imagery, metaphor, 13–14, 66, 97, 107
Immune system
    hypnotic enhancements, xvi, 75–76
Index finger attraction method, 174–75, 198
Induction imagery, 13–14, 66, 97, 107
    descending stairs, 66, 97, 107
    special rooms, 66, 97, 107
    waterfalls, 66, 97, 108
Induction process (*see* Hypnotic induction)
Infection and hypnosis
    reduced incidence, 58, 68, 85, 100
Information processing and surgical anesthesia, 59–63, 107, 120–21
Intensive care unit, 119–24
    major surgery
        bowel and bladder functioning, 73, 82, 84, 102, 113, 119
        hypnotically prepared and narcotic needs, 84, 102, 119
        intubation and appliance tolerance, 119
        nausea, 40, 82, 102, 113, 119, 120
        pain tolerance, 84, 113, 120
        relaxation, 119
    pediatric intensive care unit, 151–54
    unconscious
        hypnotic relaxation procedures, 122–24
        indirect communication input, 58, 65, 120
        information processing, 59–63, 107, 120–21
        nonverbal response mode, 120
        state of altered consciousness, xiii, 4, 6, 58, 65, 120
        suggestibility, 58, 120
International Society of Hypnosis, 20
Irritable bowel syndrome, 39, 64

L

Labile accessibility, 18

M

Manifestation of unconscious mind, 4
McGill Pain Questionnaire, 49
Medical modality, xii, 31–53
    biofeedback and hypnosis, 38, 39
    bone marrow transplant patients, 40, 41
    burns, xii, 38, 44, 102, 138
    cancer, 38, 44
    fibromyalgia, 39, 44
    invasive procedures, 97
    irritable bowel syndrome, 39, 64
    migraine headaches, 39, 44, 76
    obstetrics, 163–209
    temporomandibular disorder, 39, 40
    tension headaches, 39, 44
Memory
    comatose and information encoding, 60, 107, 120–21
    consciousness re hearing and imprinting, 60
    critically ill and information encoding, 60
    surgical anesthesia and information processing, 59–60, 107, 120–21
Mesmer, Franz A., xi, xiii, 3, 6, 99
    animal magnetism, xi, 6, 99
Mesmerism, 6, 99
Minnesota Multiphasic Personality Inventory, 165
Multiphasic Pain Inventory, 49
Multiple cognitive pathways, 5

N

Narcotics, contraindicated, 102
Nausea, emesis, 40, 82, 102, 113, 119
Neodissociation, special process theory, xiii, 5
Nonintentional vs. intentional response modes, xiii

O

Obstetrics and gynecology, 163–209 (*see also* Postpartum depression; Posttraumatic Stress Syndrome)
    amnesia, 170
    association, 170
    benefits of hypnosis, 166

Subject Index

childbirth scenario and PTSD formation, 169–71
endometriosis, 209
group vs. individual therapy, 166–67
gynecology and hypnotic session methodology, 192
   preinduction overview, 192–96
      seeding, 196
      session final comment, 209
   session 1: self-hypnosis preparation, 196–99
      age regression, 198
      environmental awareness, 198
      index finger attraction, 198
      internal awareness, 199
   session 2: special place of bliss, 199–206
      induction transcript, 200–6
   session 3: symptom specific suggestion, 206–8
      four-finger technique, 207
      glove analgesia, 207
      vocals vs. verbals, 208
hyperamnesia, 170
hyperanalgesia, 170
hyperassociation, 170
hypnotic ability and phenomena, 171–72
literature
   Handbook of Hypnotic Suggestions and Metaphors, 209
   Trancework, 208
   Uncommon Therapy, Psychiatric Techniques. . ., 186–87
normal and abnormal labor understanding, 167
physiology and psyche, 182–209
   conscious/subconscious influence, 183–96
      anorexia, bulimia re hypnotizability, 191
      defensive mechanisms re pregnancy, 191
      infertility and stress' influence, 191–92
      limbic-hypothalamic tract functioning, 189
      overview, 183–86
      physical changes re intercourse for women, 186–88
      gender of child influences, 190
      hypothalamic hormones, 188
      menstrual cycle and hormones, 188
      neuro-hormonal changes re frequent intercourse, 188
      orgasm, psychologically-induced, 189
      pituitary hormones, 188
      psychological changes via physiological factors, 188–89
   psychoneuroimmunology (PNI), 182–83, 208–9
      hysterectomy word derivation, 182–83
      hysteria, 183
      and hypnosis by definition, 183
      mind-body united complex, 182
postpartum depression, 178–82 (*see also* Postpartum depression)
preinduction, 172
   hypnotizability assessment, 173
   therapeutic objectives, 173
PTSD from labor experience, 169–71
research findings, 164–67
self-hypnosis training, 172–82
   session 1: hypnotic trance, 174–75
      index finger attraction method, 174–75
      therapeutic objectives, 175
   session 2: imagery, 175–76
      age progression, 176
      amnesia, 175
      catalepsy, 176
      hallucinations, 176
      ideosensory responses, 175
      prenatal bonding, 176
      therapeutic objectives, 176
      time distortion, 176
      transition labor phase reframing, 176
   session 3: anesthesia, 176–78
      analgesia, glove, 177–78
      dissociation, 176–77
      therapeutic objectives, 178
   session 4: reinforcement, 178
      ego-strengthening, 178
      posthypnotic suggestions, 178
symptomatic trance, 169–71
time perception distortion, 170, 176

P

Pain management (*see also* Chronic pain)
    acute pain, 31–38, 43–45 (*see also* Acute pain; Chronic pain) acute vs. chronic pain differences, 31–38
    acupuncture vs. hypnosis, 37
    biofeedback vs. hypnosis, 38
    cancer, terminally ill, 38
    case studies
        physician surgery
            breast lumpectomy, gatekeeper's thumb, 212–14
            inguinal herniorrhaphy, 216–22
        psychological significance of injury experience, 33
        Vietnam land mine injury, 32–33
    color of pain, 49
    dental patients, 38–39
    descriptive techniques, 49
    early learning experiences and transient pain, 33–34
    hypnosis and change, 37
    hypnotic techniques, 49–51
    hypnotic vs. placebo analgesia, 34–38
        hypnotizability and pain tolerance, 35–37
        ischemic pain tolerance, 34, 35
    key questions to evaluating pain patients, 47
    medical modalities and hypnosis, 38–41
    pain threshold, 34
    patient choice as to when to control pain, 51, 65
    phantom pain, 33
    sensory and affective components, 32
    shape of pain, 49
    stress inoculation vs. hypnotic analgesia, 37, 38, 83
    surgery and intraoperative recovery suggestions, 60–62
    pain management, 60
    table: adjunctive use of hypnosis in pain treatment, 42
    ——hypnotic techniques for pain control, 52
    ——key questions for evaluating pain patients, 47
Pain, perception of, 83
Pain reduction (*see also* Glove analgesia; Self-hypnosis)
    and imagery techniques, 13–14
    chronic pain, xvi, 3, 4
    ideomotor movement response procedure, 24–26
    pain sensations, organic and psychogenic, 82
    positive, negative hallucinations, 15
    postoperative pain, 3, 82–84
    psychological meaning, 83, 100
    stress, fear, anxiety management, 83
Patient coping styles
    anxiety, anger reduction,
    social control and hypnosis, 8, 65–68
Placebo response, 9–10
Positive, negative hallucinations, 15
    pain management, 15
Post Natal Major Depressive Disorder Scale, 179
Postoperative pain
    postoperative medication, 3, 58–60
    recovery time, 3, 59–60, 101–3
Postpartum depression, 178–82 (*see also* Obstetrics and gynecology)
    attributional style analysis, 180–82
        permanency, 180
            impermanent for bad, 180
        personal, 180
            impersonal bad, 180
            personal good, 180
        pervasive, 180
            nonpervasive bad, 181
            pervasive good, 181
    cognitive thinking, reframing, 179
    incidence, 178
    overview of symptoms, 179
    Post Natal Major Depressive Disorder Scale, 179
    psychoneuroimmunology, 182–83
    psychosocial factors, 179
    skill-based approach, 181
        characteristics of training program (list), 181
Posttraumatic Stress Syndrome, 17, 169
    from labor experience, 169–71
Premedication, contraindications, 102
Psyche and physiology, 182–209
    conscious/subconscious influence, 183–96
        anorexia, bulimia re hypnotizability,

191
  defensive mechanisms re pregnancy, 191
  infertility and stress' influence, 191–92
  limbic-hypothalamic tract functioning, 189
  overview, 183–86
  physical changes re intercourse for women, 186–88
  gender of child influences, 190
  hypothalamic hormones, 188
  menstrual cycle and hormones, 188
  neuro-hormonal changes re frequent intercourse, 188
  orgasm, psychologically-induced, 189
  pituitary hormones, 188
  psychological changes via physiological factors, 188–89
  psychoneuroimmunology (PNI), 182–83, 208–9
  hysterectomy word derivation, 182–83
  hysteria, 183
    and hypnosis by definition, 183
  mind-body united complex, 182
  Uncommon Therapy, Psychiatric Techniques..., 186–87
Psychoneuroimmunology (PNI), 182–83, 208–9
  hysterectomy word derivation, 182–83
  hysteria, 183
    and hypnosis by definition, 183
  mind-body united complex, 182
Psychopathological phenomenon, 7
Pulmonary complications, reduction, 85, 97, 102

R

Rapid indirect induction techniques
  four-finger technique, 207
  hypnosis and EEG patterns, 13
  hypnosis vs. sleep EEG patterns, 13
  index finger attraction method, 174–75, 198
  induction by eye roll relaxation, xi, 8, 20–26, 96, 105, 107, 133
  relaxation induction, xi, 8, 12–13, 20–26, 49, 52, 69, 97, 119, 104–41, 122–24, 133
Reflex sympathetic dystrophy, 44

Relaxation
  active alert hypnosis, 13
  four-finger technique, 207
  hypnosis and EEG patterns, 13
  hypnosis vs. sleep EEG patterns, 13
  index finger attraction method, 174–75, 198
  induction by eye roll relaxation, xi, 8, 20–26, 96, 105, 107, 133
  relaxation induction, xi, 8, 12–13, 20–26, 49, 52, 69, 97, 119, 104–41, 122–24, 133
Salivary immunoglobulin A and hypnotic induction, 60
Seeding therapy, 196
Self-hypnosis, xv, 8, 49, 64, 110 (*see also* Relaxation)
  eye roll relaxation, xi, 8, 20–26, 96, 105, 107, 133
  four-finger technique, 207
  glove analgesia, 12, 49, 52, 66, 97, 108–10, 207
  index finger attraction method, 174–75, 198
  relaxation induction, xi, 8, 12–13, 20–26, 49, 52, 69, 97, 119, 104–41, 122–24, 133
Sleep EEG patterns, 13
  alpha, beta, theta, delta waves, 13
Social-cognitive interaction, 4
Social control and hypnosis, 8, 65–68
Society of Clinical and Experimental Hypnosis, 20
Socio-psychological, cognitive-behavioral theory, xiii, 4
Special place of bliss imagery, 199–206
Special state of consciousness, 4
Stanford Hypnotic Susceptibility Scale: Form C, 7, 19, 105
Stress inoculation vs. hypnotic analgesia, 37, 38
Subcortical communication, 67
Suggestibility, form of, 4, 7
  pain reduction, 4, 10–12, 31–53, 149
Suggestion, power of, xv, 7, 10–12
  intraoperative suggestion and recovery, 58–62
  pain treatment, 12, 31–53
  pediatric surgical patients, 138–61
  physiological influences, xv, xvi, 31–53

postoperative suggestion and recovery, 57–87, 62–68, 101–3, 149
psychological influences, xv, 31–53
Surgery (*see also* Anesthesia, general; Anesthesia, regional; Hypnoanesthia)
  anesthesia, perceptions, imprinting, 59–62
  anesthesiologist's role in allaying fear, 63–64
  bleeding control, xvi, 3, 64, 72–73, 78–80, 101
  hypnosis, anxiety reduction, postoperative recovery, 57–87, 101–3
  hypnotic complications, contraindications, 67
  physiological benefits of hypnoanesthesia, 101–3
  psychological preparations, xiv, 58–87, 100
  recovery via hypnosis, physiological signs, 84–85, 101–3
  surgical conversations and unconscious imprinting, 60–62, 72
Terminology prohibitions
  almost over, 96
  finished soon, 96
  it's all over, 61
  pain, 84, 113, 120, 141
  put to sleep, 61
Trance logic, 14–15
  tolerance for logical inconsistencies, 14–15
Trance markers, 9
Trance state and protective state, ix
Trancework, 208
Trauma memories, access via hypnosis, 4

U

Unconscious
  comatose and information encoding, 60, 107, 120–21
  critically ill and information encoding, 60, 107, 120–21
  hearing and imprinting information, 60, 107, 120–21
  ideomotor movement response procedure, 24–26, 52, 60, 63, 121
  levels of, 5
  surgical anesthesia and information processing, 59–60, 107, 120–21
Unconscious motivation, 7
Unconscious processes access via hypnosis, 4

V

Venipuncture and/or venous access, 138

W

Wound healing, 58, 68, 100, 102

ABOUT THE AUTHOR

Lillian E. Fredericks, M.D. trained in anesthesiology at Hahneman Hospital and Medical College in Philadelphia, Pennsylvania and practiced at the Albert Einstein Medical Center in Philadelphia, where she was Chief of the Department of Anesthesiology during the Second World War. This was followed by an appointment to the Department of Anesthesiology at the Hospital of the University of Pennsylvania, where she practiced for more than seven years, until her retirement. Dr. Fredericks started a twelve-weeks course in Medical Hypnosis at the University. She is a Diplomat of the American Board of Anesthesiology, Diplomat of the American Board of Medical Hypnosis, Fellow American Society of Clinical Hypnosis, Fellow American Society of Clinical and Experimental Hypnosis, Fellow International Society of Hypnosis, and Fellow Swedish Society of Clinical Hypnosis. Dr. Fredericks is a Member of the World Medical Association and listed in *Marquis Who's Who in Medicine*. In 1995, she received the Shirley Schneck Award for Significant Contributions to the Development of Medical Hypnosis, given by the Society for Clinical and Experimental Hypnosis. Dr. Fredericks has given several papers and workshops during the yearly meetings of all the societies mentioned above. At present, Dr. Fredericks is in private practice and still busy preparing for future talks.

Publications

Fredericks, L.E. (1942). Prevention of shock in spinal anesthesia. *The American Journal of Surgery, 56*(2), 438–445.

Fredericks, L.E. (1958). Oxygen saturation during hypotensive anesthesia. *Journal of the Albert Einstein Medical Center, 6*(2), 100–104.

Fredericks, L.E. (1961). Anesthesia for patients with jaundice. *American Journal Gastroenterology, 36*(1), 44–50.

Fredericks, L.E. (1963). Pheochromocytoma. A Conference of the Cardiology Department, Albert Einstein Medical Center. Volume 11, 211–13.

Fredericks, L.E. (1981). Hypnosis in Pediatrics. Lecture given at The Philadelphia Society of Clinical Hypnosis. Published in Philadelphia Medicine.

Fredericks, L.E. (1966). *Anesthesia for open heart surgery.* Springfield, Illinois: Charles C Thomas.

Fredericks, L.E. (1967). The use of hypnosis in hemophilia. *American Journal of Clinical Hypnosis, 10*(1), 52–55.

Fredericks, L.E. (1978). Teaching of hypnosis in the overall approach to the surgical patient. *American Journal of Clinical Hypnosis, 20*(3), 175–183.

Fredericks, L.E. (1980). The value of teaching hypnosis in the practice of anesthesiology. *The International Journal of Clinical and Experimental Hypnosis, 28*(1), 6–14.

Fredericks, L.E. (1982). Alternate methods of anesthesia. *Dangerous Properties of Industrial Materials Report. 2*(4), 6–15.

Fredericks, L.E. (1988). Hypnosanesthesia and preparation for surgery. 30th Annual Scientific Meeting and Workshop in Clinical Hypnosis, Chicago, IL.

Charles C Thomas
PUBLISHER • LTD.

P.O. Box 19265
Springfield, IL 62794-9265

A Leader in Behavioral Sciences Publications!

- Brooke, Stephanie L.—**TOOLS OF THE TRADE: A Therapist's Guide to Art Therapy Assessments. (2nd Ed.)** '04, 256 pp. (7 x 10), 19 il., $53.95, hard, $35.95, paper.

- Moon, Bruce L. & Robert Schoenholtz—**WORD PICTURES: The Poetry and Art of Art Therapists.** '04, 246 pp. (7 x 10), 44 il.

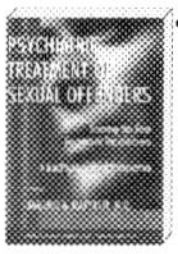

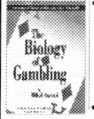

- Aasved, Mikal—**THE BIOLOGY OF GAMBLING. Volume III.** '04, 372 pp. (7 x 10) $86.95, hard, $57.95, paper.

- Aiken, Lewis R.—**MORALITY AND ETHICS IN THEORY AND PRACTICE.** '04, 300 pp. (7 x 10), 31 il., 9 tables, $65.95, hard, $46.95, paper.

- Cruz, Robyn F. & Cynthia F. Berrol—**DANCE/MOVEMENT THERAPISTS IN ACTION: A Working Guide to Research Options.** '04, 250 pp. (7 x 10), 7 il., 9 tables, $58.95, hard, $38.95, paper.

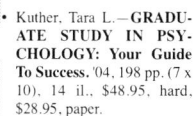

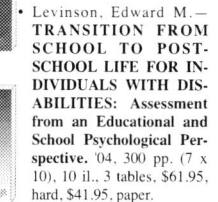

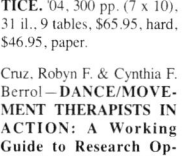

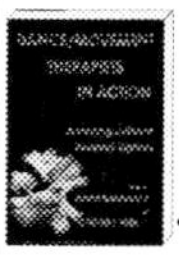

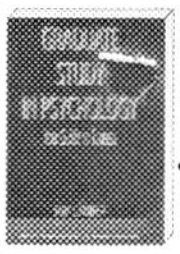

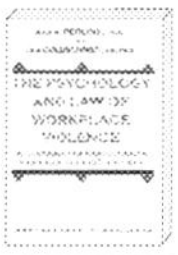

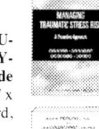

- Kuther, Tara L.—**GRADUATE STUDY IN PSYCHOLOGY: Your Guide To Success.** '04, 198 pp. (7 x 10), 14 il., $48.95, hard, $28.95, paper.

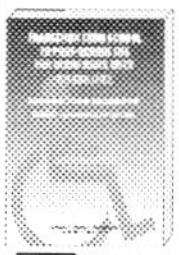

- Levinson, Edward M.—**TRANSITION FROM SCHOOL TO POST-SCHOOL LIFE FOR INDIVIDUALS WITH DISABILITIES: Assessment from an Educational and School Psychological Perspective.** '04, 300 pp. (7 x 10), 10 il., 3 tables, $61.95, hard, $41.95, paper.

- Marvasti, Jamshid A.—**PSYCHIATRIC TREATMENT OF SEXUAL OFFENDERS: Treating the Past Trauma in Traumatizers-A Bio-Psycho-Social Perspective.** '04, 220 pp. (7 x 10), $49.95, hard, $34.95, paper.

- Marvasti, Jamshid A.—**PSYCHIATRIC TREATMENT OF VICTIMS AND SURVIVORS OF SEXUAL TRAUMA: A Neuro-Bio-Psychological Approach.** '04, 234 pp. (7 x 10), $53.95, hard, $33.95, paper.

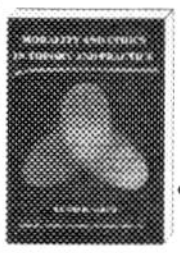

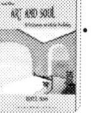

- Moon, Bruce L.—**ART AND SOUL: Reflections on an Artistic Psychology. (2nd Ed.)** '04, 184 pp. (6 x 9), 15 il., $44.95, hard, $28.95, paper.

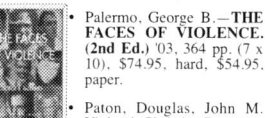

- Palermo, George B.—**THE FACES OF VIOLENCE. (2nd Ed.)** '03, 364 pp. (7 x 10), $74.95, hard, $54.95, paper.

- Paton, Douglas, John M. Violanti, Christine Dunning, & Leigh M. Smith—**MANAGING TRAUMATIC STRESS RISK: A Proactive Approach.** '04, 258 pp. (7 x 10), 6 il., 17 tables, $61.95, hard, $41.95, paper.

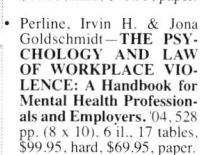

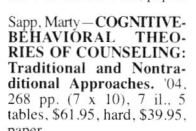

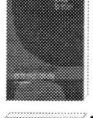

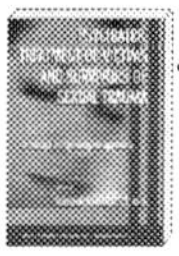

- Perline, Irvin H. & Jona Goldschmidt—**THE PSYCHOLOGY AND LAW OF WORKPLACE VIOLENCE: A Handbook for Mental Health Professionals and Employers.** '04, 528 pp. (8 x 10), 6 il., 17 tables, $99.95, hard, $69.95, paper.

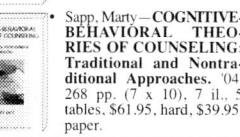

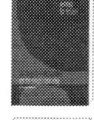

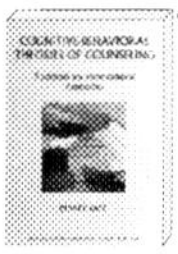

- Sapp, Marty—**COGNITIVE-BEHAVIORAL THEORIES OF COUNSELING: Traditional and Nontraditional Approaches.** '04, 268 pp. (7 x 10), 7 il., 5 tables, $61.95, hard, $39.95, paper.

- Donahue, Brenda A.—**C. G. JUNG'S COMPLEX DYNAMICS AND THE CLINICAL RELATIONSHIP: One Map for Mystery.** '03, 302 pp. (7 x 10), 15 il., $64.95, hard, $44.95, paper.

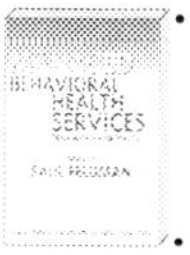

- Feldman, Saul—**MANAGED BEHAVIORAL HEALTH SERVICES: Perspectives and Practice.** '03, 460 pp. (7 x 10), 6 il., 10 tables, $77.95, hard, $57.95, paper.

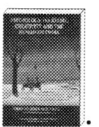

- Heuscher, Julius E.—**PSYCHOLOGY, FOLKLORE, CREATIVITY AND THE HUMAN DILEMMA.** '03, 388 pp. (7 x 10), 3 il., 1 table, $53.95, hard, $33.95, paper.

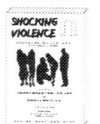

- Moser, Rosemarie Scolaro & Corinne E. Frantz—**SHOCKING VIOLENCE II: Violent Disaster, War, and Terrorism Affecting Our Youth.** '03, 240 pp. (7 x 10), 1 il., 4 tables, $49.95, hard, $32.95, paper.

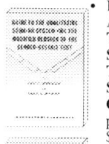

- Brannigan, Gary G. & Nancy A. Brunner—**GUIDE TO THE QUALITATIVE SCORING SYSTEM FOR THE MODIFIED VERSION OF THE BENDER-GESTALT TEST.** '02, 154 pp. (7 x 10), 49 il., 6 tables, $37.95, hard, $24.95, paper.

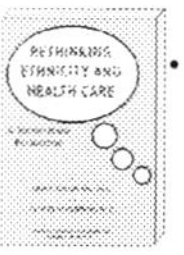

- Ma, Grace Xueqin & George Henderson—**ETHNICITY AND SUBSTANCE ABUSE: Prevention and Intervention.** '02, 360 pp. (7 x 10), 1 il., 10 tables, $75.95, hard, $53.95, paper.

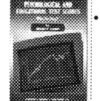

- Sapp, Marty—**PSYCHOLOGICAL AND EDUCATIONAL TEST SCORES: What Are They?** '02, 204 pp. (7 x 10), 3 il., 21 tables, $49.95, hard, $31.95, paper.

5 easy ways to order!

PHONE: 1-800-258-8980 or (217) 789-8980
FAX: (217) 789-9130
EMAIL: books@ccthomas.com
Web: www.ccthomas.com
MAIL: Charles C Thomas • Publisher, Ltd. P.O. Box 19265 Springfield, IL 62794-9265

Complete catalog available at ccthomas.com • books@ccthomas.com

Books sent on approval • Shipping charges: $6.95 min. U.S. / Outside U.S., actual shipping fees will be charged • Prices subject to change without notice